face VALUE

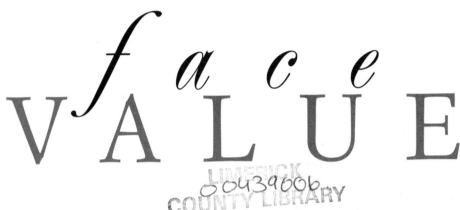

face VALUE

The Truth about Beauty— and a Guilt-Free Guide to Finding It

HEMA SUNDARAM, M.D.

A Living Planet Book

RODALE

© 2003 by Hema Sundaram, M.D.

Interior photgraphy © by Digital Vision/Getty

Printed in the United States of America
Rodale Inc. makes every effort to use acid-free ∞, recycled paper ♻.

Book design by Christina Gaugler

Library of Congress Cataloging-in-Publication Data

Sundaram, Hema, M.D.
  Face value : the truth about beauty—and a guilt-free guide to finding it / Hema Sundaram.
      p.   cm.
  Includes index.
  ISBN 1–57954–708–7 hardcover
  1. Women—Health and hygiene.   2. Beauty, Personal.   3. Face—Care and hygiene.
I. Title.
RA778.S9295   2003
646.7'042—dc21   2003005776

Distributed to the book trade by St. Martin's Press

2   4   6   8   10   9   7   5   3   1   hardcover

For my daughter, Vidya, whose face is beyond value

She walks in beauty, like the night
Of cloudless climes and starry skies;
And all that's best of dark and bright
Meet in her aspect and her eyes . . .
　　　　　　　—Lord Byron

Acknowledgments

My heartfelt gratitude and thanks go to the following people:

Joshua Horwitz of Living Planet Books, for his friendship, insight, encouragement and inimitable "magic touch" throughout the whole process of writing this book.

Gail Ross, my agent, for her infallible professional advice.

The talented and dedicated team of professionals at Rodale, my publishers, especially Mary South, for seeing a diamond in the rough and acquiring this book; Mariska van Aalst, my editor, for polishing that diamond to a fine sheen; and Christina Gaugler, my designer, for setting it so beautifully.

My husband, Gopal Srinivasan, for his love, support, encouragement and friendship not only during the writing of this book, but also throughout our fourteen years together.

My children, Vidya and Giridhar Srinivasan, for the joy, laughter and transcendent beauty they have brought to my life; with special thanks to Vidya for her enthusiastic reading and critique of my drafts.

My parents, Saroja and Trichur Sundaram, who have always made me feel beautiful, selflessly supported me in every endeavor, and taught me that the most important aspect of beauty—and life—is balance.

My friend, Cindy Snyder, and my professional colleague and friend, Dr. Patricia Walker, for their thoughtful reading and critique of my early drafts.

My wonderful staff—Mirvia Arroyo, Rania Elbashir, Dahlia Hassan, Taj Hassan, Deepa Subramanian and Vasanthi Vittal—for their skills, professionalism, loyalty and team spirit, for making each day at the office a pleasure . . . and for uncomplainingly picking up the slack during my long months writing this book.

And finally, my patients, the inspiration for this book, from whom I have learned—and continue to learn—so much.

Contents

Introduction

When I was just a little girl
I asked my mother, "What will I be?
Will I be pretty? Will I be rich?"
Here's what she said to me:
"Que será será,
whatever will be, will be. . . ."

—as sung by Doris Day

My favorite song as a toddler—the one my mother had to sing to get me to eat my cereal—often rings in my ears these days when I'm talking to patients in my dermatology office. I think it's because Doris Day's 1950s anthem of equanimity neatly encapsulates the defeatist attitudes that many women have toward beauty even today. The entire mindset is there: our deepest desire, from early childhood, to be beautiful and our indoctrination with the fatalistic attitude that destiny alone determines whether or not we achieve beauty. After all, Doris suggests, there's little we can do about it except wait and see.

I've never had a patient yet who came in humming the strains of "Que Será Será," but I've met many whose refrains sounded remarkably similar. Take Beth, who is 39 and tells me, "I guess I just wasn't cut out to be anything more than cute." Or Andrea, in her fifties, who sighs, "My sister was always the beautiful one."

How many women these days declare that they are simply not destined to be intelligent, or successful in their careers, or good mothers? We don't relinquish control over any other aspect of our lives except beauty. And we don't denigrate those who aspire to any other attribute the way we do those who quest for beauty.

We position beauty and intelligence as polar opposites, as if by definition a woman's IQ must be inversely proportional to her looks. And we save our most strident condemnation for those who choose to enhance their beauty through cosmetic surgery, labeling them traitors to the cause of feminism, shallow and vain. In doing so, we ignore one simple fact: *We are evolutionarily programmed to seek beauty because that's what keeps the human race going.* Put a 5-year-old in a room with a fabric remnant and a wisp of netting, and she'll turn it into a dress-up outfit. Why, then, should we be surprised when a 50-year-old also wants to look her best?

Finding My Own Face Value

This book is about face value. Not just in the literal sense, the value we all place on superficial appearance whether we care to admit it or not. But also in another sense: the importance of understanding what truly gives *your* face its value. True beauty has both inner and outer aspects. You can attain your fullest face value only if you understand how to surface your inner beauty in your face and wed it harmoniously with your outer beauty. This book will show you how.

My path to discovering my own face value was part of what inspired me to write this book. My background straddles several cultures. I was born in America, the daughter of two Indian émigrés, but grew up and was educated in England. I'm now a cosmetic dermatologist living and working in the suburbs of Washington, D.C.

As one of the few non-white students in my British school, I often felt different-looking and at odds with the prevailing standard of beauty. That's why I can readily empathize with anyone who feels the same way.

My path to discovering my own face value took almost two decades. It started in my pre-teen years. That's when I became acutely aware that how I looked didn't conform in any way, shape or form to how the media—the books and magazines I read, the TV programs I watched, the girl-talk swirling around me and so on—told me I "should" look. I was different. And that can be a devastating discovery at an age when your overwhelming preoccupation is with "fitting in."

But I came to appreciate with time that being different, deviating from the norm, can actually be an advantage. It was a sudden realization that sparked this appreciation. I'd always loved wordplay; cryptic crosswords and literary brainteasers were my favorite amusement from childhood onwards. And, as I was studying a crossword puzzle one day in my mid-twenties, it occurred to me that being "abnormal" and being "extra-ordinary" are really two sides of the same coin. After all, both mean that you are not normal, that you're out of the ordinary or different. But how much more uplifting and empowering it is to view oneself as extraordinary, rather than as abnormal!

Luckily for me, the Hindu culture within which I was raised helped me to transcend the dualities, the two-sided coins, that characterize so many of the dilemmas women face about their physical appearance. Mind and body, male and female qualities, love and sex, science and spirituality, were always presented to me as integrated life forces, not warring factions. Specifically, inner and outer beauty were always understood to be a continuum, with beauty originating in your soul and finding expression in your body. The stages of life were also viewed as a continuum, and the body as an evolving mirror of your soul's spiritual development.

I think it's vital for every woman to appreciate this continuum. Because we're all different—maybe not as dramatically as I was with my dark hair and skin amid a sea of rosy schoolgirl complexions—but different nonetheless. And there is one cultural differentiator we're *all* destined to acquire with time. To age is to be quintessentially different in a society which pushes youth as the norm and as the ultimate hallmark of beauty. I believe that we can only cope successfully with the changes of aging if we've already accepted being different as a positive attribute. This means redefining our concept of beauty, to make it more individual, inclusive and holistic.

I don't preach to my patients, and I'm certainly not promoting Hinduism. What I *am* advocating is a woman's right and ability to follow whatever path to beauty she chooses, at any age, without guilt, shame, or judgment.

My Relationship with My Patients

At my British medical school, I was taught that there is a unique bond between physician and patient. When a patient permits a doctor to lay hands on her, it is the greatest honor that the doctor can receive. I am still mindful of this today, every time I enter an exam room and meet a patient, whether for the first or the 50th time. I've always considered my patients to be equal partners in whatever treatment plans we formulate.

Much of this book is based on what I have learned from my patients over the years. My relationships with my patients extend beyond cold, clinical confines to encompass a level of trust and intimacy that I believe has few parallels in other medical fields. The nature of my work is part science and part art, but I am frequently also confessor and psychologist to my patients. They confide in me regarding the daily events of their lives and often ask my advice.

I see and hear firsthand how women suffer as they age, and I witness the integral connection between events of the soul and external events. This intimacy has allowed me to develop a deeper understanding of the psyches of women. I study faces and body language in my office every day and can often tell a lot from them: who is happy and who is not, who has inner peace and who does not, who has a desire for change and who does not. Most important, I've been able to learn which attitudes are most likely to achieve a positive result—that is, feeling as good as you look—and which are counterproductive or downright destructive.

I would not have chosen the field of cosmetic dermatology and remained in it if I were not utterly convinced of the positive effects of cosmetic surgery performed for the *right* reasons. One of the joys of my profession is seeing on a daily basis how restoring the balance between a woman's inner and outer selves can transform her life.

My relationship with my patients is collaborative, and they have a high level of input into the treatment plans I devise for them. I have learned that no two patients have the same patterns of aging or the same objectives, and thus these treatment plans must be carefully individualized to achieve optimal results. This book is drawn from my experiences in trying to help women of all ages and backgrounds look and feel their best.

I've illustrated many of the points in this book with anecdotes based on my experiences with my patients. In these anecdotes, their names have been changed to protect their privacy. And in some cases the stories are based on more than one patient.

My Program

During our initial consultations, my patients often pose the million dollar question of beauty: Can a woman slow her rate of aging?

Yes, you can retard your rate of aging, and I'll show you how in this book. But, more important, I'll offer you a holistic prescription for harmonizing your inner and outer beauty and, I believe, for finding authentic empowerment in midlife.

This book recognizes that your inner and outer beauty are inseparably linked and shows you how to develop them together. My step-by-step integrative beauty regimen includes lifestyle changes that will retard aging and enhance your beauty; an up-to-date and honest appraisal of at-home skin rejuvenation and in-office cosmetic procedures; meditations that are specifically designed to develop and project your inner, spiritual beauty; and much more. I'll also show you how you can enhance your external beauty by whatever means you decide are right for you, including cosmetic surgery.

I wrote this book for every woman who has ever looked in the mirror and felt betrayed by the passage of time—or by what she thinks time will inevitably take away. It's a guilt-free guide for any woman who has contemplated cosmetic surgery and been tormented—or puzzled—by her own conflicted feelings or by conflicting messages from others. It's for every woman who wants to find a sane middle ground between a relentless youth culture and her natural desire to slow the aging process. And it's written for, and dedicated to, every woman who recognizes that her desire to be beautiful and to *stay* beautiful is perfectly natural.

I'm going to give you the same information, trust, encouragement, and freedom to choose that I offer all my patients. And I hope that this program will help you to recognize and achieve your *own* face value.

part one

Beauty Is Truth
and Truth Is Beauty

chapter one

Tackling Our Taboos
about Beauty

Youth is something very new;
twenty years ago no one mentioned it.

—Coco Chanel

eauty has been headline news lately. We've heard all about Greta Van Susteren, the cerebral news reporter and lawyer who shocked the nation by having very obvious cosmetic surgery on her very public face. We've read about Botox parties, where guests join their hostess for conversation, canapés—and a few shots in the forehead to iron out their frown lines. And then there's actress Jamie Lee Curtis, who showed up in literally nothing but her underwear—unstyled, un-made-up, unmasked—in *More* magazine. Showing us her real, unadorned, imperfect self, Curtis confessed to having had cosmetic surgery and vowed penitently never to do it again.

Even the traumatic events of the past couple of years have done nothing to dampen our fascination with all things cosmetic. The tragedy of September 11, 2001, severely damaged our economy, but the media were full of reports about how it didn't decrease the number of cosmetic procedures performed. In fact, many cosmetic surgeons found that their patient visits actually *increased*. The theory? When people are thrown into a situation of stress, despair, and powerlessness, they seek to control what they can—in this case, their appearance.

I vividly remember my astonishment that terrible day as virtually all of my patients still showed up for their appointments even as I was desperate to leave the office, collect my children, and go home to wait for news of missing family members. In the ensuing days, I even had calls from patients who were not scheduled to see me, wondering if I "might have an opening today because of what happened." As my assistant, Taj, wryly commented, if we had ever doubted the power of the human drive to be beautiful, we would never do so again.

I want to talk about that drive, and the chase it creates. The media tell us that both the drive to be beautiful and the chase for beauty are politically incorrect; and that women are victimizing or debasing themselves by giving in to them. And we all get infected by this negativity. We deny Van Susteren's intelligence because she succumbed to their blandishments. We praise Curtis for coming clean (or we question her timing, noting that she sang a different tune when she was starting out in Hollywood and establishing her reputation as "The Body"). And we voyeuristically scoop up the gossip about Botox parties, eagerly looking for disasters among the vanity. There's no doubt about it; cosmetic surgery is good copy.

Underscoring the dictum that there really is no such thing as bad publicity, Van Susteren, Curtis, and the myriad talking-head doctors opining about Botox all have done very well for themselves plumbing the depths of our fascination with beauty, cataloguing the extent of what human beings will do to their faces and bodies in its pursuit. It's high-profile because it evokes high emotion in most of us.

And that's why, as a female "beauty doc," I meet few people who are indifferent to what I do for a living. As a rule, I instantly polarize whatever room I walk into. I'm manna from heaven to women who want the skinny on what's new and hot in the world of cosmetic surgery. And I'm a traitor to the cause to others, who view cosmetic surgery as a latter-day abomination dredged up from antifeminist hell.

The reason for this polarization is that women are in conflict. We're simultaneously exhorted to be beautiful and condemned for the means we use to achieve that beauty. It's worth keeping in mind that cosmetic surgery is only the latest focus of that conflict. A few generations ago, we felt the same way about makeup, and we labeled women who wore it as fast and loose. And in mid-1970s England, when I was about 11, hair spray was the focus!

On the one hand, I remember one television advertisement that told women that beauty was all. Josephine, the mistress of the French emperor Napoleon, was making her way through the pouring rain to the battlefield tent of her lover. But by the time she reached him, her once-immaculate coiffure was wet and bedraggled. He uttered the immortal line "Not tonight, Josephine," and advertisers extolled the benefits of their hair spray in preventing your hair from "letting you down."

The other side of the coin was the archetypal 1970s beauty striding down the street, her long, blond hair flowing behind her, with every passerby asking the same question: "Is she or isn't she?" This question was eventually revealed as pertaining to hair spray, and the up-front message was clear: if you were using something this unnatural, it had better be undetectable. (The subliminal message was equally clear in the moralistic double entendre of "Is she or isn't she?")

You may recall this British advertisement's latter-day American descendent; it hawked hair coloring with the slightly modified double entendre, "Does she or doesn't she?" Note that coloring your hair—unlike spraying it—is directly related to aging. Such was the extent of our "progress": we moved from impugning beauty enhancement in general, to impugning *age-related* beauty enhancement in particular.

It seems ludicrous now that we would ever imply, even subliminally, that hair spray or a dye job make you immoral. And, indeed, we've moved beyond that now . . . to a *new* emblem of morally suspect vanity: cosmetic surgery.

When you think about it, beauty and beauty enhancement are about the only aspects of our lives where we still tolerate being judged, or feel it's still socially and politically acceptable to be judgmental about others. Gone, after all, are the days when you could condemn a woman for having sex or having a job or having a vote. But, rather than let go of these supposedly obsolete judgments, it seems that we've merely redirected them.

The huge irony of all this is the part the women's movement has played in this redirection. Women are living in an era of ever-expanding social and professional vistas, and we've all benefited from the women's movement. It's encouraged us, and enabled us, to seek parity in every aspect of our lives. And it's liberated us from many attitudes that held us back from fulfilling our true potential. It's ironic that the instrument of our liberation has imprisoned us in one basic respect—by making us feel it's wrong to want to be beautiful or to want to stay beautiful as we get older . . . particularly if we seek medical intervention to do so.

Can a Feminist Get a Face-Lift?

We portray those who seek medical intervention as victims of some modern-day scourge and denounce that intervention as a backlash against feminism. Think of how Jamie Lee Curtis is cast in the role of victim, symbolically stripped of her defenses when she's vulnerably stripped to her skivvies.

In fact, cosmetic surgery is as old as the hills. Chemical peeling has been around for aeons, and nose jobs and fat injections were happening even a century ago. What's different now is that we have more efficient technology for making ourselves over, and this gives us better and safer results with less recovery time.

Are women at risk of becoming victims of cosmetic surgery? Of course we are—just as we're at risk of becoming victims in relationships, the workplace, and every other facet of our lives. But I believe the focus shouldn't be on censorship, but on educating women about the true nature of beauty and the right and wrong reasons to have cosmetic surgery. After all, there's nothing to be achieved by acting like a Victorian English father at the breakfast table, reading aloud to his wife and children only the newspaper articles he deems acceptable for their ears.

Listen to real women who've had cosmetic surgery performed well and for the right reasons. They don't sound like victims at all. Take Jennie, who told me, "You've made it fun for me to wear lipstick again," after I filled in the puckered lines around her mouth with collagen. She defined her fun on her own terms. Or Anne, a recently widowed 53-year-old, who used cosmetic surgery to help herself cope with the stress of her husband's death and the toll it took on her appearance and self-image.

Cosmetic surgery can take advantage of us only if we let it. It's insulting and patronizing to women to suggest that it should be condemned wholesale because of this, as if it were the Eighth Deadly Sin. The outrage vented upon those who choose to make use of this technology reminds me of the behavior of the Luddites. They decried as immoral the factory machines that threatened their livelihood, and they destroyed them. Now some people are using their moralistic opinions to smash at what threatens *them*. It's a horrifying thought, but pinning the label of "shallow traitor to the feminist cause" on a woman who has cosmetic surgery is really no different than hanging a scarlet letter around her neck.

Take my patient Ilene, who wanted three undesired moles removed from her face but was insistent that this didn't count as cosmetic surgery.

"I wouldn't have it done if it was," she declared emphatically. "I don't know why people mess around with all those machines and chemicals," she continued, sweeping her hand through the air over her face. "They ought to be stopped."

Remember yourself as a small girl, pirouetting without self-consciousness in front of a mirror in your first dress-up clothes? Now think of what we're doing to ourselves. We've taken the fun out of being beautiful—and we've replaced it with guilt.

Fear, Anger, Shame—for What?

I want you to step back from all this polemic and ask yourself one question: In a country that wrote the book on freedom of the individual, why do we condemn those who have had, or wish to have, cosmetic surgery?

I think one reason is that we're afraid. I'm not talking about the fear of surgery itself—that you'll meet your medical Nemesis in the form of a death or injury if you indulge. Nor am I talking about the fear that inept surgery will leave you looking like a parody of yourself or, worse, a parody of a Barbie doll. (Although I can well understand this fear when I see a movie star with an appallingly bad face-lift or lopsided collagen treatment.)

What I'm talking about is a much more basic fear—the fear of death. We transfer a lot of the fear and anxiety we feel about death to the issues of beauty and beauty enhancement. We do this because, in a society which sees beauty and youth as synonymous, aging is the ultimate reminder of our mortality and the harbinger of our deaths. Seeking cosmetic surgery is an admission that physical beauty, although transient, is important . . . and also an admission that we are aging, mortal beings who will eventually die. We speak of cosmetic surgery in moralistic terms and label it as evil, but underlying this is our feeling, to paraphrase Socrates, that the greatest evil is death.

There's some anger mixed in with the fear too—anger that by signaling youth they don't possess, women who have cosmetic surgery are at an unfair advantage and are operating under false pretenses. Now, if I make your friend from high school look 10 years younger than you with some strategically placed Botox and a little laser surgery, you could argue that that *is* false pretense. But then, so are push-up bras and mousse that makes your thinning hair look fuller and high-heeled shoes that round your rump—none of which we condemn with anything like the vitriol we reserve for the woman who's had her face or her breasts done.

In fact, in today's world, that anger is unfounded. Cosmetic surgery is definitely an advantage (if it's performed well), but it's no longer unfair because it's no longer the preserve of the rich or famous. One company is fond of saying that Botox treatments two or three times a year won't cost you any more than the tally of your daily cup of coffee and bagel.

You might be amazed at who's having cosmetic surgery these days. My patients come from every walk of life. They certainly include "ladies who lunch," but they also include ladies who *make* lunch, like Sandi, who works at a local deli. Sandi is neither rich nor famous, but, as she tells me, "I'd rather spend my money on my face than on a vacation—a vacation is over quickly, but my face is with me forever."

The final emotion in the cosmetic-condemnation cocktail is shame. In an era when sexual guilt seems, on the surface, so quaint and old-fashioned, we've sublimated that repressive emotion into guilt about the desire to preserve our beauty. Beauty and sex are directly and intimately related. The value and significance we place on beauty are only social side streets off the main road of an essential biological truth: The purpose of beauty is sex and the reproduction that results from it.

Look at how we react to cosmetic surgery—the furtiveness when we ourselves do it, the prurient interest when we suspect someone else did, and the way we tear apart the Jezebels who brazenly reveal all they've done. If it sounds hauntingly familiar, that's because it all directly parallels how we previously reacted to women's having sex.

No More Backroom Botox

When these three emotions—fear, anger, and shame—govern our reactions, we thrust a woman who would enhance her beauty into one of three roles: the Victim, the Cheat, or the Harlot. In doing so, we push cosmetic surgery underground, and *this* is what actually makes women victims because it often leads them to bad decisions. When I see a woman spend less time and effort choosing the surgeon into whose hands she'll place her face than she does selecting a cantaloupe in the supermarket, I get very alarmed. But that's what shame and guilt will do to you. That's how we devalue the fate of our faces.

If you want to find a good OB/GYN or a reputable dentist, you probably call a few girlfriends and ask them in detail about the doctor they go to and whether they're happy. But how many women feel comfortable doing that where cosmetic surgery is concerned? And even if they do, how many women know what questions to ask? Most end up relying on word of mouth without getting all the information they need to make an informed choice, on advertisements in the media, or on those "best doctor" lists in local magazines. If you're lucky, any of these may yield the perfect cosmetic surgeon for you. But who wants to bring luck into a decision like this?

To complicate matters further, we not only demonize cosmetic surgery—we also deal with our discomfort by trivializing it. We refer to these important medical and consumer decisions as "a little nip and tuck." And now there's the bizarre phenomenon of Botox parties, as if choosing to have cosmetic surgery were no different from choosing a piece of Tupperware.

The media's portrayal of women who have cosmetic surgery is telling evidence of our emotional baggage. These women are victims, kooks, or often both. Think of the HBO series *Sex and the City*. The outrageous, promiscuous Samantha has a chemical peel, which she blithely describes as "an impulse purchase." (Apparently, women who have casual sex also indulge in casual cosmetic surgery.) Of course, Samantha lives to regret her sin when she's forced to attend a fancy party looking like a burn victim and her fellow guests recoil in horror. Or remember Goldie Hawn's crazy character in the movie *The First Wives Club*, having her lips pumped up like demented balloons at her own behest? Or Brenda Blethyn's character in the movie *Lovely & Amazing*, who goes into the hospital for a little bit of liposuction (so, as she says, "I can feel better about myself") but slips into a coma and wakes up in excruciating pain. Where's the example of the woman who escapes beauty enhancement with her dignity intact?

Freeing Beauty from the Glass Box

In my years of practice as a cosmetic dermatologist, I have often pondered the old saying that beauty is the first present nature gives to women and the first it takes away. When I think of the dilemmas women face regarding their physical appearance as they get older, I think of the age-old tale of Snow White.

We all know the story: Snow White is the beautiful princess who's murdered by her vain stepmother queen and entombed in a glass coffin. Why does this brutal folk tale endure as a perennial favorite among children and parents alike? I believe it's because the story tells us something profound and timeless about the ongoing struggle within each of us: between youth and age, between innocence and loss, between vain, skin-deep beauty and a beauty that transcends aging.

Snow White also speaks volumes about our culture's conflicted view of beauty and its pursuit by women—about how society's adulation of youthful beauty kills with kindness, draining women of life and its psychic complexity, objectifying them and placing them on display, just like Snow White in her transparent glass box. At a young age, we're taught the hopeless lesson that beauty is at once beloved and hated by others and can survive only in suspended animation—an untouchable, sexless state incompatible with real life. And when we're unlucky enough to graduate to the role of the aging queen, we risk being viewed as vain, envious, and angry.

Virtually all the fairy tales we were raised on featured aging women as shriveled crones, objects of fear and contempt. It's no wonder that women seem to view the approach of menopause as a sword of Damocles waiting to drop randomly on their heads. The dread is made worse by fear of the unknown. It's only recently that women have even begun to talk to each other about menopause.

It's sobering to realize that menopause has been irrelevant for most of the 300 or so generations of human existence. In the past, a woman had little chance of reaching this milestone and, if she did so, less chance of being in good health. If she was lucky, she might be revered for her wisdom, but all too often, she was feared for her abnormal longevity and branded a witch—or an evil, bitter crone.

Midlife is clearly a time of significant change for women—physically, psychologically, and spiritually. The challenge facing each of us is how to make this transformation a positive and enriching one, rather than a nightmare scenario of self-contempt.

Twice-Born Beauty

We've come a long way in recent years toward recognizing menopause and perimenopause—the 10 or so years that precede menopause—as important life passages that have the potential to transform a woman's life in a positive way. Many women speak of menopause as an experience of rebirth or an entry into a new stage of life. It is a time for taking stock of life, for embarking on new personal or professional journeys, or for beginning a spiritual quest. And we have a new awareness that midlife is just that—the middle of our lives. A woman entering menopause today has half her life still ahead of her and every expectation that this will be worthwhile and productive.

I firmly believe that midlife is also an opportunity for the rebirth of your beauty, both inside and out. This might seem paradoxical since the impending end of fertility and the accelerated rate of skin aging around the time of menopause can make a woman feel less attractive. As my patient Lisa lamented, "I seem to be just sitting here, watching my face fall apart." But your face in midlife, while it may not be youthfully perfect, reflects the confidence, self-esteem, and self-acceptance that develop from life's experiences. This physical manifestation of your inner beauty, derived from your soul, increases with age. *My goal is to show you how you can surface what's within you to express your beauty in a new, infinite form that transcends the effects of aging.*

The concept that spiritually developed individuals are "twice-born" appears in many religions, including Hinduism and Christianity. The initial physical birth is followed, at any stage in life, by a spiritual rebirth. Hindu philosophy likens this to the life of a chick, which is born once within an egg and then twice-born when it hatches through the shell.

I want you to think about the next few years of your life as a period of beauty rebirth. You can use this time to develop your twice-born beauty; a harmonious combination of your spiritual and physical aspects, as tender and unencumbered by the baggage of your old expectations and outdated beliefs as the first, tentative steps of that baby chick.

The challenge of reviving beauty is to take a fresh look at yourself, relocate your beauty—both internal and external—and figure out how to renew it in a timeless form that will flourish throughout your life. And it *is* challenging because we're conditioned to see youth as beauty and age as loss.

Surfacing the Beauty from Within

We divide beauty into many artificial categories—natural and unnatural beauty, outer and inner beauty, politically correct and politically incorrect beauty. These dichotomies confuse and conflict us and pit us against one another. They make us grow unhappy as we age. In the end, if we don't figure out our own definitions for beauty, they conquer us.

No cosmetic regimen, procedure, or surgery alone is going to magically turn back the clock and restore your youthful beauty. I've watched all kinds of women pursue beauty for all kinds of reasons, and there's one consistent pattern: If you're using cosmetic procedures or surgery to please someone else, rather than yourself, or because you feel that being more beautiful will automatically make you happier, you're not going to be satisfied with the result. And you won't be happy either if you're using cosmetic surgery to chase the mirage of your lost youth.

Cosmetic procedures can repair the wrinkles and sun damage, but they can't make you truly beautiful unless you also project beauty from within. And they can't stop time. What they can do is make you look as good outside as you feel inside—provided you also *work* at feeling good inside. Otherwise, you're not escaping your glass box—you're just trading one box for another.

When I talk about feeling good inside, I'm not talking about fixing every emotional problem, whether it's a bad relationship or an underdeveloped sense of self. To me, inner beauty is something we all possess—the trick is to recognize it and build it up, rather than focus on what we lack. It's a parallel process to cultivating outer beauty—building on strengths rather than focusing on weaknesses.

With this in mind, let's revisit Jamie Lee Curtis and her magazine spread. What exactly is it that makes her a victim? She says her procedures didn't work because they didn't make her feel happier or more beautiful. But what's more relevant is that she was pushed into cosmetic surgery by others who told her she "needed" it because she wasn't good enough as she was. Curtis says that she didn't feel comfortable with herself and has suffered in the past from feelings of inadequacy. I don't think it's fair to blame these negative emotions on cosmetic surgery; after all, they pre-dated the surgery by a long while. I'm not surprised in the least that Curtis' surgery never made her feel beautiful. She had it for the wrong reasons. Using examples like hers to condemn cosmetic surgery wholesale is akin to claiming you should never eat because food can make you fat, or you should never use computers because they might crash.

Believe this: We all have inner beauty. You don't have to solve every problem in your life to express your inner beauty; you simply have to rec-ognize it and reclaim it. I've seen just how beautiful women can become when they manage to surface their inner beauty in their faces. If I con-vince you of nothing else, I want you to believe that you don't have to look like a magazine cover girl to be beautiful. You simply have to play to your strengths and not be hemmed in by irrational conflicts about how to best enhance them. Free yourself from the world's opinions, and your inner beauty will shine for that world to see.

Beauty on Your Terms

Bottom line: I'm tired of the way the media portray women who aspire to stay beautiful as they age. I'm appalled by the way our society pits women against one another and demands that we take a political stand on beauty, which is something as elemental as oxygen. I want to help women escape the airless glass box that traps them into accepting any-thing less than the best for themselves. That's why I've written this book.

Many of my patients have encouraged me to share my approach with a wider group of people because they find it unlike any they've en-countered before. I don't believe that the program I'm offering you is the only way, because it's not—there are many ways. The key is to find the approach that's right for *you*. I want to help you develop your own personal strategy for beauty.

You'll notice this book doesn't have one of those A-to-Z formats that give you basic information on all your options. There are many excellent books already available for you to consult, if that's what you want. I *will* give you information about points of interest on the cosmetic surgery map, but I'm more concerned with giving you a constructive strategy for getting what you want from this map than with charting out the entire map itself.

The primary step in developing your overall strategy is to understand and appreciate the beauty that dwells within you. If you want to be and stay fully beautiful, you need to understand—and really *believe*—how important it is for you to develop and project your inner beauty.

Then, you can take the next step toward learning how to make informed, rational decisions about what you want to incorporate into your beauty program and what you don't. Separating your true wishes from the messages that have been foisted upon you is no easy task, but it is essential. Otherwise, any shame, anger, or fear may cause you to make ill-considered decisions based on a desire to avoid criticism—from society, your friends, or even your doctor.

As you progress, you'll learn how to master certain situations with confidence. If you decide to consult a physician—whether a cosmetic dermatologist, a plastic surgeon, or a surgeon of another specialty—you need to know how to choose the right one for you, what questions to ask, and how to make informed decisions about what you want from this physician. You also need to know how to judge if you're ready for cosmetic surgery—by which I mean whether you have the optimal mindset to get the results you want.

From what my patients tell me and from what I've observed myself, the typical cosmetic surgery consultation begins with the doctor's asking you, "What do you want to fix?" or, worse, with the doctor's telling you, "This is what *I* think you need to fix." But this is putting the cart before the horse. The first question your doctor should be asking you—and you should be asking yourself—is "Why are you here?"

Ideally, your doctor will help you choose what's right for you only after she first understands you. Why, at 30, do you feel like your face is suddenly betraying you? What motivated you, at 40 years old, to visit a cosmetic surgeon? Why are you, at 50, taking action against the frown lines you've had for decades? You cannot always count on your physicians to ask these questions and explore them with you—and that's why you need to know the answers *yourself*.

As a dermatologist with an academic background in genetics, I've always been fascinated to observe how your skin is the nexus of all factors affecting beauty, from your spiritual being to your pheromones, your genetic imprints to your lifestyle. If, as the poets say, the eyes are the windows to the soul, then surely your skin is its mirror. If you're stressed-out, angry, or depressed, your skin will telegraph it to the world. If, on the other hand, you are at peace with yourself, your skin will radiate contentment.

But recognizing your inner beauty and the impact it can have on your whole persona is only half of the equation. For many women, the most distressing part of the aging process is that their faces no longer project their image of how they feel inside. Puffy, drooping eyes make a face look tired; frown lines prompt passers by to wonder, "What's she so angry about?" Thin, wrinkled lips can convey sadness, even when none exists. As my patient Anne put it, "My face has become my enemy."

The landmarks of life, such as turning 40 or reaching menopause, may cause you to scrutinize your appearance more carefully and to become more aware of the changes of aging. "This is a quality-of-life issue," my patient Lisa told me. "The wrinkles bother me more now, and it's more important to me to fix what I can."

When what you project externally no longer evokes a positive reaction from others or yourself, this inevitably impacts how you feel internally. You look in the mirror and feel that the outer image does not truly represent who you are inside. This mismatch between your inner Self and your outer persona is, to me, the correct reason to consider cosmetic surgery.

There is an old Hindu saying that we pass through life in a stupor, blinded by external distractions from seeing the truth within us. But even though you are not aware of your inner self, it is awake and ever present. At life's end comes the inevitable realization: "I was never a dreamer, but was always awake." Don't wait—let this be your wake-up call to the ageless beauty burning within you. Feed the fire, make it blaze, and ignite your beauty!

Bewitched by Beauty

*Nothing makes a woman more beautiful
than the belief she is beautiful.*

—Sophia Loren

*L*et's be honest: We all want to be beautiful and sexually attractive. It's nothing to be ashamed of—it's how we're wired, genetically and culturally. Women have beautified themselves since time immemorial in pursuit of both biological and social success.

Despite this age-old imperative, I've discovered that most of my patients in midlife are conflicted about their desire to improve their appearance, even those who are in situations where it's vital to project a youthful, energetic persona. Recently, for instance, Helen, a dynamic and highly successful realtor in her forties who routinely brokers high-profile transactions, looked me straight in the eye and told me, "You have to get rid of my wrinkles so that I can keep my edge." Yet only a few minutes later during the consultation, she averted her gaze from me and whispered, "My husband and colleagues would be shocked if they knew I was doing this." Another of my patients, Lisa, was concerned that "You must think I'm incredibly vain, but you've got to help me."

I'm confronted with this paradox on a daily basis. Women know that their appearance is usually the first thing others notice about them and that this can have a profound effect upon their personal and professional interactions. They spare no effort to enhance their appearance and self-esteem through dress, a good haircut, and makeup. As they enter midlife, they become aware of, and seek to stave off, the changes wreaked by the aging process. But they feel guilty about doing so, especially about expressing the wish to have corrective cosmetic surgery. They are concerned about how others will perceive them—even I, the physician they are consulting for this surgery! Most of all, they're afraid of being labeled "vain." It's no wonder we end up in the glass box of self-consciousness, self-contempt, and guilt. Forget about the glass ceiling—I'm talking four impregnable, suffocating walls!

Why do individuals who are quite uninhibited in expressing their needs and desires in other arenas find it so difficult to do so when it comes to improving their appearance through cosmetic surgery in particular, or even to pursuing beauty in general? Why does the prospect of being thought vain strike so much fear in otherwise stalwart hearts?

I think it begins with us—with women's history, with our biology, with our gains in equal rights and with our own knee-jerk reactions.

We've been indoctrinated with the notion that the pursuit of beauty and cosmetic surgery are modern inventions thrust upon Western women in an attempt to subordinate them as they gained liberation. But history and evolutionary science belie this polemic. In fact, it's altogether natural that many women in midlife want to take steps to retard the physical evidence of aging and to enhance their beauty.

Midlife can be your escape hatch from the glass box. Instead of seeing this stage through the prism of fading youth or "Over the Hill" birthday balloons, you have to start appreciating the gifts of this stage; you have now amassed the unassailable confidence, self-esteem, and self-acceptance that develop from life's experiences. This appreciation gives your inner beauty—which is derived from your soul and increases with age—the opportunity to flower so that you can finally break out of the stereotypes that box you in.

Many women entering midlife are engaged in a quest for inner beauty. These days, this may be through conventional spiritual means, such as yoga, or simply through finding activities that inspire them toward self-acceptance. If you want to truly embrace your freedom to stay beautiful, the first challenge is to develop your inner beauty. The second is to surface that inner beauty, project it and unite it with your outer persona. And also to improve upon what's outside, if you wish.

I'm not advocating that every woman should rush out and have cosmetic surgery as soon as she notices her first wrinkle. It's your choice whether or not you wish to enhance your outer beauty. And, if you do, it's up to you whether you do it through lifestyle modifications, at-home skin care, cosmetic surgery, or a combination of all three. If something bothers you, fix it. If it doesn't, leave it alone.

But what I am advocating is the right of every woman to make this most personal decision herself. And I don't believe this decision should be influenced by anger, shame, or fear of what others might think.

Midlife—the most profoundly transformative passage of your life—is your opportunity to reclaim your birthright: beauty in its fullest and most timeless form. The precise formula for expressing this beauty is yours, and yours alone, to determine.

The Fleeting Gift of Youthful Beauty

To truly understand why the glass box limits us, we must begin at the beginning—in childhood. When we look at our children, the beauty of youth seems effortless and everlasting. But when taken in context of an entire lifetime, that perfect youthful beauty is as fleeting as morning dew.

Watch those children at play, and you will be struck by the unconscious and un-self-conscious beauty of youth. When my daughter, at 7, tossed her head and told me, "I'm beautiful because of my hair," and my 4-year-old son giggled with delight at his image in the mirror and kissed it, they didn't attach any stigma to the desire to be beautiful. Children appreciate the importance of being beautiful and often derive great pleasure from it. And they're not afraid of being considered vain.

Children also don't view aging in a negative light. They aspire to be older and look up to their elders. I'll never forget driving my daughter and her two friends home from drama class when they were in kindergarten. The three girls were competing to see whose mother was the oldest. I could only imagine the looks on the faces of the other two mothers had they been there to witness the conversation. It was a real—and hilarious—eye-opener to see how differently young girls, and the women they become, view the aging process.

What happens to this connected and effortless beauty as we pass from childhood into adulthood? Somewhere along the line, we become increasingly aware of prevailing standards of beauty and others' reactions to our appearance. We become aware of comments that are made about us and start to define ourselves in terms of the way we are perceived. By young adulthood, we've all acquired labels: "the pretty one," "the red-head," "the one with good hair," "the one with bad skin." Of course, we're acutely aware of these labels, we internalize them, and we begin to define ourselves by them. In effect, we're complicit in allowing these labels to reduce us from three-dimensional human beings to two-dimensional clichés.

Many of my patients describe treading this path of self-consciousness and self-doubt in their young adult lives. Close your eyes and think back to the effortless beauty of your youth. There it was, in all its glory, but did you ever really appreciate it at the time? Or were you fixated on all the flaws you thought you had, assuming that they were all everybody else would see?

Comments about our appearance often remain with us—and sometimes scar us—for life. I vividly recall complimenting a friend's looks in medical school, only to see her shake her head firmly in denial, reliving the teenage memory of her aunt's telling her mother, "But you are so beautiful—how could you have such an ugly daughter?" Or I think of my college friend, who refused at the last minute to attend a party with me because she had run out of base makeup and was convinced that if others glimpsed her bare skin, they would be horrified by its imperfections.

When I think back to my teens, I can still feel my own uneasy sense that I didn't conform to anyone's ideals of beauty. In my largely white high school, I was acutely aware that my brown skin and black hair made me stand out—and who wants to stand out when she's a teenager? I was told that my black hair looked "dirty," and a classmate whom I hardly knew wrote a teasing note about my lips in my graduation booklet. I threw the booklet in the trash can, rather than take it home.

Compounding matters was my feeling that I did not epitomize Indian beauty either—my face was too angular, my hair too wavy, and my eyes the wrong color to emulate the oval-faced, sloe-eyed, sleek-haired woman idealized in India. I was frequently described as "exotic," but I didn't really take this as a compliment—it put me in the same category as a white tiger at the zoo. The only compliment that did mean something was the one I received from my father in my late teens. Perhaps sensing my thoughts, he told me that I had an "interesting" face.

The judgment of a harsh world, and the even harsher judgment we inflict upon ourselves, mire us in self-consciousness and self-contempt. As a result, we no longer bare our souls to the world, but wall off our inner, childlike beauty from our outer, physical beauty. The wall serves something of a protective function: it shields our deepest souls from the barbs of a critical world.

And so we find ourselves in the glass box, on passive display to a world that rates us by its objectified standards of external beauty, in a contest we can never win. If you're one of the "lucky" few, you're judged to be beautiful. You may be adored for this, but you're simultaneously reviled. You are so defined by your appearance that it often seems as though the rest of you has become a mere appendage of your beauty—generally overlooked and unappreciated.

Hiding Your Peelings

Women today are subjected to a merciless barrage of conflicting messages about the universal drive to look our best at any age. We should always look great, but never be vain. We owe it to ourselves to do whatever we can to look younger, but not ever let anyone know how we're doing it. And whatever beauty regimen we follow, it had better be "natural."

On one hand, the media celebrate youth and sexuality. They promote beauty as an absolute virtue, along with an endless stream of anti-aging "cures." At the same time, women are made to feel guilty about any beauty regimen that crosses the divide between "natural" and "artificial."

No wonder we feel conflicted! We're bombarded with images that tell us youth is a prerequisite for beauty. Every magazine cover reinforces an objectified standard of beauty—which is usually computer-enhanced and therefore unreal—as the ideal. But society tells us to strive for this through "natural" means!

Some cosmetic procedures carry no stigma at all, but procedures that are most directly related to aging do. If it is not "wrong" for a 14-year-old to straighten her teeth orthodontically, why is it "wrong " for a 40-year-old to have laser surgery to remove her wrinkles? Eyebrow shaping, if done artfully, and pierced earrings, if well-chosen, can profoundly enhance a woman's looks and even appear to alter the contours of her face. But they don't engender guilt; why, then, should liposuction of a double chin? Why don't we feel ashamed of having manicures and acrylic nails, which drastically alter the "natural" appearance of our hands?

A number of women have suggested to me that it's the money involved, but it's obviously not. Any harried parent of a teenager can attest to the fact that braces often cost more than extensive laser surgery. Furthermore, a nose job costs about the same whether it's performed for cosmetic or medically necessary reasons. But I've lost count of the patients who rush to assure me that their nose jobs were not for mere vanity. Christie is typical, pointedly telling me, "The doctor said the nasal surgery might improve my breathing. I just asked him to smooth out the bump as a secondary thing."

Why do *People* magazine's "50 Most Beautiful People" extol the beautifying virtues of their exercise regimens, their spiritual pursuits, and their hobbies but never acknowledge the role of cosmetic surgery—even when it's patently obvious? What drives Cher to swear *on her children's lives* that "I've never had ribs taken out, cheek implants or anything like that"? And what drives the media to push her into this guilty denial? Even Britain's staid, sober—and liberal—*Observer* newspaper gets in on the act, asking Goldie Hawn what she's "had done" and being met with this stonewalling response: "Okay, I'll tell you what I have had done. I had under my eyes done. And that was it." Clearly, cosmetic surgery arouses intense emotional conflict in women . . . and in those who judge them.

We think of some types of beauty enhancement as natural or corrective, and hence acceptable, and others as unnatural or "cosmetic," and hence unacceptable or sinful and to be hidden at all costs. A glance at the health and beauty section of any bookstore reveals this prevailing doctrine. Woman are exhorted to embrace the natural and to avoid the unnatural. Cosmetic surgery is considered to be the epitome of unnatural—and thus sinful—beauty enhancement.

But the concept of distinct "natural" and "artificial" methods of beauty enhancement is nonsensical. If you massage your face with common table salt at home, it's considered a natural beauty remedy. If I polish your skin in my office with the same substance (sodium chloride) to remove wrinkles or discolorations—a procedure known as salt macro-dermabrasion—this procedure is labeled as "artificial."

I believe that the viewing of anti-aging cosmetic surgery as a sin is merely a reflection of the fact that we view aging itself as a sin. Just as one can be on the "right" or "wrong" side of 40, so one can use the "right" or "wrong" methods to obviate aging—with cosmetic surgery's being the ultimate "wrong" method. In one brochure advertising collagen implants for the treatment of wrinkles, a woman says: "We all agreed to age gracefully. Then we found out some of our friends were cheating."

We have been conditioned to think of aging and anti-aging strategies in moralistic terms: good and bad, honest and cheating. The new beauty dogma states that "good girls don't have cosmetic surgery," an ordinance every bit as constraining as those to which women were subjected in the past in the name of morality.

Beauty behind Closed Doors

Maybe Freud had it right—everything does come back to that most elemental of acts. I'm convinced that our conflicts about the explicit pursuit of beauty are rooted in our society's mixed feelings about sex. On one hand, we live in a hypersexualized, ostensibly "liberated" culture. At the same time, we have a deeply moralistic, even puritanical, streak that judges the pursuit of sex, and by extension of beauty, as morally suspect—particularly when it's a woman in midlife who's doing the pursuing.

Social critics, both male and female, have demonized cosmetic procedures as politically incorrect and dangerous. Ten years ago, in *The Beauty Myth*, Naomi Wolf made no bones about her impression of the beauty industry, describing "invasive potentially deadly 'cosmetic' surgeries" as "permanent, painful, and risky alteration(s) of the body."

In fact, cosmetic surgery has never been safer, more effective, or more widely available than it is now. We live in an era when cosmetic surgery is increasing exponentially in popularity. I mentioned one of the primary reasons for this increase earlier: the advanced technology that allows us to achieve better results, often with shorter recovery time. Interestingly, two other reasons for the increase in cosmetic surgery are directly linked to an increase in women's power: a steady rise in women's discretionary income and a dramatic shift in the way we view the middle years—as the prime of life rather than preparation for death. What would Wolf make of the supposedly subjugating nature of women's beauty decisions in light of these reasons for the industry's growth?

Recent advances in the safety and effectiveness of cosmetic procedures—such as laser resurfacing, Botox, liposuction, and face-lifts—as well as their increased popularity would seem to belie their enduring stigma. But as with sex, we prefer to do our cosmetic surgery behind closed doors and talk about it only among our close friends, if at all, and we feel guilty or ashamed when exposed by the media—or judgmental and titillated when others are exposed.

You may have noticed that now there is also a subset of patients who do the opposite and they flaunt the "work" they've had. Some social critics hold this up as evidence that we're now comfortable with cosmetic surgery. But let's draw the sexual analogy again: is the woman who boasts of her sexual conquests in all their explicit detail any less insecure than the woman who furtively hides all?

Look at the front-page coverage of Greta Van Susteren's recent makeover. Here's a woman, struggling to keep pace in the mercilessly competitive field of broadcast news, who can admit neither that her cosmetic surgery was premeditated ("I did it on a whim") nor that it was extensive ("I just wanted to take a few dents out"). Is this liberation? Or does it remind you of women of the 1950s explaining away sexual encounters with the excuse that "It just happened" and downplaying how far they went?

And look how the media reacted to Van Susteren's surgery, first by "outing" her to an outraged public and then by questioning the credibility of her intellectual image. One newspaper report began with the Neanderthal "Duh . . ." and the suggestion that Van Susteren could no longer be taken seriously, given what she'd had done.

The reaction in on-line chat rooms was even more savage. Van Susteren in particular, and cosmetic surgery patients in general, were excoriated for being shameful, pathetic, devoid of all self-respect, and traitors to the cause of feminism. Cosmetic surgery was decried as an abomination that morphs its victims into plasticized monstrosities, and Van Susteren was held up as the prime example.

Ultimately, Van Susteren was absolved in the modern-day confessional. In her front-page story in *People* magazine, she "frankly" and "fearlessly" told all (or as much as she wanted to tell), titillating us sufficiently for us to grant her redemption.

Van Susteren discovered that the glass box can be a cold and lonely place that only heightens our need for acceptance. We're torn between the desire to look beautiful and the fear of what others—our friends, our colleagues, our families, our "sisters"—will think if we are seen to be trying too hard. Over the past half century, this desire to conform to a specific standard of outer beauty has been blamed upon societal (particularly dominant male) pressure.

In *The Beauty Myth*, Naomi Wolf presented the politically correct view that "for about 160 years middle-class educated Western women have been controlled by various ideals about female perfection." She laid the blame for this at the doorstep of the beauty industry and other male-dominated institutions. This is not realistic.

The truth is, we've had ideals of female perfection since antiquity. In some respects, the details have changed. The thin-lipped, high-browed, consummately Caucasian beauty of medieval Europe has yielded to a more voluptuous and ethnically inclusive facial stereotype. Yet we should remember that the hallmarks of female beauty are based upon sound evolutionary principles. Beauty and our appreciation of it are important and always will be, no matter if it's unfair, politically incorrect, or guilt inducing.

The Evolutionary Role of Beauty

When a beautiful face turns our heads, we're responding to incontrovertible evidence of fertility, good genes, and willingness to mate. This evidence made visible defines a beautiful female face. When we see clear skin that is free of blemishes and male-distributed facial hair; long, thick, shiny hair; and white teeth, we see a persuasive evolutionary advertisement: youth, plentiful estrogen and good health, and consequently fertility. (This link is vividly illustrated by the disease polycystic ovary syndrome, in which cysts on the ovaries cause a hormonal imbalance, with lowered estrogen levels. This results in acne, unwanted hair—and concomitant infertility.)

Other criteria of female beauty signify sexual arousal. Think of large eyes with dilated pupils, full red lips, and flushed rosy cheeks—all with the inherent promise of sexual receptivity, successful mating and reproduction. But perhaps the ultimate proof of beauty that originates inwardly but is expressed outwardly is the existence of pheromones.

The pheromone has enthralled us since it was first discovered in insects, decades ago. The much-debated human version has aroused tremendous excitement in the scientific community, and no wonder. What other substance could you produce internally and release into the air to completely alter other people's perceptions of you, entirely without their knowledge?

There's another, equally intriguing group of related chemicals known as "odor quality signals", which differ from true pheromones chiefly because they have detectable smells, whereas pheromones do not. In the discussion below, I'm going to use the term "pheromone" generically, to refer to true pheromones and also to odor quality signals. That's because much of the research in this field doesn't distinguish between these two types of chemical signals.

The reputation of pheromones as stealth messengers of sexual attractiveness has given rise to a slew of spray-on products supposedly laced with animal pheromones, which claim to make you "irresistible to those you desire!" One pheromone perfume manufacturer was recently reported to be raking in revenues of more than $40 million per year. The scientific basis of spray-on "pheromones" is definitely shaky. After all, the whole point of pheromones is that they are exquisitely specific even within the same animal species, so it's highly unlikely that a human being could be aroused by what gets a goat's motor going. But what's driving this business is the compelling truth of what we *do* know. Pheromones and similar chemical signals control every aspect of animals' lives—how they grow, with whom they mate, and how they raise their offspring. What remains to be proven is whether pheromones control human lives, down to and including our perception of beauty.

The suggestions are provocative. Have you ever been inexplicably drawn to someone—male or female—regardless of or out of all proportion to physical appearance or personality? Perhaps you have had your emotions stirred, or long-lost memories evoked, by a simple odor—like the smell of your partner's shirt or your child's hair? Have you ever noticed that your "privacy zone"—the distance you feel comfortable keeping between yourself and another person—varies quite markedly according to who that other person is? When we speak of having good or bad "chemistry" with someone, we are literally—and scientifically—quite correct. Chemicals *are* important in determining whom we find attractive and whom we don't.

One pheromone study introduced the compelling possibility that beautiful women may indeed have it all—including the best pheromones. This study, done by Rikowski and Grammer in Austria, found that women whose photographs were judged by men to be more attractive and whose faces were more symmetrical on the basis of specific measurements were also judged to have more highly rated body odor, based on how their tee shirts smelled after being worn for 3 consecutive days.

We have a long way to go to understand the complex interplay between the primal instincts driving our appreciation of beauty. Jutte, another Austrian researcher, found that men seem to care more about body odor when they are evaluating a woman whom don't they find particularly attractive visually—and they rate her beauty more highly if they like what they smell. Perhaps this is Mother Nature's way of showing us beauty *is* more than skin deep; appealing pheromones may compensate to some extent for a plain face.

Evolution comes into play when we consider that we may inherit our body odor preferences. One study done by Swiss researchers, Wedekind and Furi, at the University of Bern, suggests that we tend to prefer the body odors of people who are genetically dissimilar to us. The offspring of two genetically different individuals often have an evolutionary advantage. Think of hybrid vigor, the phenomenon by which a plant produced from two genetically different plants is often healthier and more resistant to disease than either of its parents. When we're drawn to those different from ourselves, perhaps we are increasing the odds of robust progeny. Could it be that our vision of beauty is actually rooted in our biological sense of the person whose genes would give our offspring the best chance of survival?

I offer this argument as yet more proof that we haven't begun to fully understand the role of beauty in the survival of our species. To dismiss a powerful instinct that's helped perpetuate humankind for hundreds of thousands of years as a mere political ploy cooked up to subjugate women just seems a bit short-sighted, doesn't it?

Beauty of History, Myth, and Legend

Beyond the world of science, the universal importance of beauty is seen across time and cultures and is reflected in some of our most powerful literature and myths. The "smallest" of these stories—fairy tales—actually wield tremendous influence upon our opinions, norms, and expectations. Like so much else, our first notions of beauty are imbibed on our mothers' laps.

Think, for instance, of Rapunzel, whose long hair "as fine as spun gold" was ample testament to her estrogen status; or of Snow White, with her skin "as white as snow," cheeks "as rosy as blood" and hair "as black as ebony." Indian stories dating back 1,000 to 5,000 years describe "long, thick hair black as a rain cloud, soft and glossy, with a billowy curl," teeth "like a string of pearls," and "large eyes like the black bee moving in the petals of the lotus"—a simile that blatantly and directly invokes the vision of fertility.

Women have beautified themselves since the start of recorded history, beginning with the deliberate removal of facial hair and the strategic reddening of lips. Cosmetic procedures also have a long pedigree. When Cleopatra bathed in sour milk or the ladies of the 17th-century French court applied aged wine to their faces, they were treating themselves with alpha hydroxy acids, a mainstay of many modern skin-rejuvenating regimens. Medieval European women used small doses of the poison atropine to temporarily paralyze and dilate their pupils; the other name for atropine is "belladonna," Italian for "beautiful lady."

Throughout history, women have found themselves subject to societal expectations and also largely powerless to seize control of their own images. To women of ancient Greece, the mythologized Helen of Troy— with a face that "launched 1,000 ships" and a divine beauty described as immune to aging—must have been every bit as intimidating as the supermodels on today's magazine covers are to us. Helen was certainly every bit as unrealistic as today's supermodels, with their computer-generated perfect skin and squares of cardboard taped to the backs of their heads to make their hair look fuller. All that's changed is that we've become more efficient at concocting and disseminating the image of perfect female beauty. But when we blame the media for stereotypical female imagery, we're simply blaming the messenger for the message.

Bewitched by Beauty

So why *do* we prize beauty and yet feel so uncomfortable about it? Both our guilt about the desire to preserve beauty and our demonization of cosmetic surgery are manifestations of our two most primal drives: sex and the fear of death.

We adore physical beauty, but it makes us incredibly uncomfortable precisely because it's so random. You can't control it; you're either "born with it" or you're not. Aging, and the fading of beauty, seems uncontrollable and reminds us on a daily basis of the inevitable and ultimate uncontrollable: We are mortal beings, and we will eventually die.

Throw in our mixed feelings about sex and the way we relate these feelings to the quest for beauty, and it's no wonder we see witchcraft in beauty and in those who pursue it. The glass box helps subdue the witchery. It takes the ultimate uncontrollable—real, living, active, multi-faceted, mortal beauty, the lightning rod for desire and envy, our most powerful and frightening emotions—and reduces it to the lowest common denominator of femaleness. We enter a passive, suspended, sexless state that is nonthreatening to society and to ourselves because it denies the inherent sensuality of beauty and the inevitability of aging.

Look at our fairy-tale heroines. They're all ageless icons, pristine in their untouchability. And they suffer for their beauty. Rapunzel is incarcerated by a wicked old witch and has her hair cut off. Snow White's aging stepmother becomes insanely jealous of her beauty and youth and attempts to destroy her. Sleeping Beauty is cursed to fall into a stupor when she pricks her finger on a needle.

Notice how Rapunzel in her tower, Snow White in her glass box, and Sleeping Beauty on her four-poster bed are enclosed in nonthreatening passivity. Although you won't catch Disney trumpeting this angle, the sexual analogies are quite obvious here, made all the more evident given that each heroine is imprisoned when on the threshold of womanhood and then "rescued" into marriage by a savior prince who "penetrates" her enclosure. The beauty message is equally obvious: we don't feel comfortable unless beauty is repressed into sexless captivity.

There's no doubt that the objectified standards of beauty imposed upon women are immensely unfair and that we all have a right to feel angry about them. But when we react by flying in the face of nature and denying the importance of beauty, we miss the point. It's not the *desire* to be beautiful that traps us. Rather, it's guilt and shame over the desire to be beautiful and the fear of what others will think because we *want* to be beautiful. Denying that beauty has always captured our imaginations only perpetuates the unfairness and the objectification. It reinforces the notion that outer and inner beauty are separate and distinct or incapable of coexisting. The premise that if you look good outside you can't have anything meaningful inside is what prevents us from enjoying or even appreciating our own beauty at any age.

The result is that we end up in a timeworn struggle, separated largely along gender lines, between those who would preserve the glass box and those who would deny its very existence. This struggle is played out vividly in art. Male literature throughout the ages has focused on female physical beauty. Think of Thomas Hardy rhapsodizing about Bathsheba, his heroine in *Far From The Madding Crowd*, for whom "...criticism checked itself as out of place and looked at her proportions with a long consciousness of pleasure." Now, pick up a male-authored novel or a male-oriented magazine from the airport bookstore and you'll see the same concept, albeit more prosaically and explicitly expressed.

The sole example I can find of male literature that appears to downplay the importance of outer physical beauty, actually bears closer inspection. Winston Smith, the protagonist of George Orwell's *1984*, gazes out a window and describes a mature woman—her figure coarsened by childbirth and her hips "a metre across"—as the fulfillment of youthful beauty. Smith is a rebel. His challenge to our generally accepted notions of beauty epitomizes his challenge to the whole infrastructure of the world in which he lives. Our tenets of beauty are so deeply ingrained that Orwell uses rebellion against them to symbolize rebellion against the whole of society.

And then there's our female literature which, in its efforts to celebrate well-developed inner beauty, tends to espouse women who do not possess conventional outer beauty. For example, Charlotte Brontë's Jane Eyre is described by her suitor as "small and plain," but with a "searching and yet faithful and generous look." Louisa May Alcott's Jo, the heroine of *Little Women*, is spirited, intellectual, and good-hearted, but she is not the prettiest sister; her one beauty is her hair which she ultimately relinquishes. The worthiness of these heroines is based as much upon their outer beauty as on their possession of inner beauty.

Deconstructing the Feminist Fallacy

I see the conflict and confusion that result from this stark dichotomy every day in my patients, in the women I meet socially, and sometimes even in my potential employees.

Rose interviewed for a position as my nurse shortly after I started my solo practice. She hadn't known before meeting me that I have a special interest in cosmetic dermatology and when she discovered this, she spent the rest of her interview asking me what could be done for her face. I've certainly had other interviewees who did the same. What makes Rose stand out is that she called the next day and said that she would love to join my office, but she explained, "I have two teenage daughters, and how could I possibly tell them where I work?" You would have thought I was running a backstreet drug dealership!

Rose's story is a perfect example of what I call the feminist fallacy, the simultaneous fascination and revulsion we feel for the beauty chase combined with an irrepressible desire to be "good" and obey the dicta of political correctness. Rose—and the rest of us—can tell our daughters until we're blue in the face that it doesn't matter how they look; that what matters is what's inside. If we're really determined, we can shield them for a brief period from anything that shatters that illusion, including books, movies, and other people. But nature will still have its way. Women will still be primping and men will still be looking at them in

1,000 years' time because that's what makes the world go 'round and our species continue to exist.

I think it's far better to be honest with our children from the outset. The worst way to damage your daughter's self-esteem is to lie to her, because then you make her feel that she's not worthy of the truth. And the truth is that outer beauty *is* important—but that's not the whole truth. The rest of the truth is that the epitome of beauty has always been much *more* than merely physical.

The ancient Hindu ideals of Satyam, Shivam, and Sundaram (truth, auspiciousness, and beauty); Plato's tenets of beauty, justice, and truth; and today's quest to be "more than just a pretty face" illustrate that beauty is of universal and timeless importance, but the most desirable beauty will always be a harmony of internal and external components. Consider that we use the oft-repeated statement "Beauty is only skin deep" to describe those who we feel possess only external physical beauty, or that the word "vain" is derived from the Latin word for "empty." Who wants to simply project an empty beauty, a shell without a core?

Even our fairy-tale beauties possessed both outer and inner beauty. Snow White was good-hearted and kind; the Indian heroine with pearly teeth was said to be "as high-souled and heroic as she was beautiful." Why is this kind of harmony so hard to believe in for living, breathing women?

Divided against Ourselves

Insisting that we separate our outer and inner beauty pits women against one another. Ironically, the feminist fallacy—the idea that you are "betraying" other women by wanting to be beautiful—perpetuates this. Let's say that despite your buying into the idea that beauty isn't important, you still fear losing your attractiveness in midlife. The feminist fallacy, by making you feel guilty about this fear, only increases your vulnerability. You don't speak out about it, because you're afraid of what your friends, colleagues, sisters will say, and voilà! The cycle repeats itself, and the walls of the glass box are reinforced for another generation of women.

My goal isn't to refute conventional feminist doctrine—the last thing we need is women slinging more mud at one another, particularly when we, as females in America, owe so much to the women's movement. Rather, I want to offer you a broader perspective on the age-old pursuit of beauty, from a scientific, evolutionary, and cultural perspective. The sooner we can liberate ourselves from our conflicts about pursuing beauty, the sooner we can start looking and feeling better. And the first step is to recognize the ideal of physical female beauty for what it is: a primeval fantasy, a prehistoric blueprint, a tantalizing promise deeply embedded in our biological and sociological DNA.

The desire to be beautiful wasn't invented by Madison Avenue or *Vogue*. We're magnetically drawn toward beauty and fascinated by what can be done to make us more beautiful. Yet at the same time, we feel uneasy and guilty about our beauty preoccupation, and we transfer these negative feelings onto those who seek beauty (including ourselves) and the methods they use—especially cosmetic surgery.

The truth is, beauty arouses more emotion than other unevenly distributed gifts, such as intelligence, precisely because we consider it to be so important. When we brand those who pursue beauty and youth as heretics to the cause of female equality and burn them at the stake of public opinion, we're no different from our forebears who demonized old age and launched witch-hunts against crones with hairy moles. Our reactions are simply a manifestation of our discomfort.

If you can make the leap beyond the punishing dichotomies I've illuminated, you open up endless possibilities for both beauty and happiness. Acknowledge your right to define your own beauty and your freedom to cultivate both its inner and outer aspects . . . and you'll be ready for true beauty at any age.

chapter three

Are You Ready to be Beautiful?

*The beauty that addresses itself to the eyes
is only the spell of the moment; the eye
of the body is not always that of the soul.*

—George Sand

If you want to formulate a winning strategy for beauty, it's crucial that you understand that your inner and outer beauty can coexist. In fact, they *must*.

Think of the handful of times in your adult life when you have felt wholly beautiful. Visualize a moment of personal triumph at home or work when your inner and outer beauty seemed completely in harmony and you truly felt and looked your best. These moments are fleeting, and you may find them becoming scarcer as you get older.

That's the downside of midlife. During your reproductive years, you're accustomed to viewing yourself through the prism of your fertility and the physical attractiveness this confers upon you. As menopause approaches, you may feel less attractive not only because your aging rate tends to increase at this time but also simply because you're confronting the end of your fertility. As we've discussed, fertility is inextricably entwined in our notions of beauty.

But there's an upside too. The wisdom, awareness, and insight of midlife can catalyze you into recognizing your inner beauty and the life force within you. You can finally reach the stage of accepting, valuing, and even celebrating your own appearance. My patient Susan recalled turning 40 as the time when "I stopped obsessing about my bad points and started to focus on my good points."

As you pass through midlife, you may discover you're ready to become beautiful in a way you've never been before, simply by letting your inner beauty lead the way. How that inner beauty will manifest itself—and the path you take to bring it to the surface—is exactly what I'm here to help you discover.

Harnessing the Power of Midlife

When you stand back from all the Madison Avenue product hype, there's no need to view midlife as the beginning of a woman's slippery slide into decrepitude. Hindu philosophy, for instance, speaks of the dynamic surge of energy that arises in a woman of middle years, originating in the base of her spine and other defined energy centers and spreading throughout her body. This surge is said to be so strong that when uncontrolled, it can shatter lives and relationships. But when harnessed positively, it can lead to inspirational and momentous experiences.

Whether you keep your wrinkles or do something about them, make sure it's your choice and not a choice foisted upon you by someone else. Also, you must rethink your concept of beauty as your externalized, fleeting youth that you hope to recapture. That way lies madness, or at least frustration.

I want you to see your beauty instead as something that you always possess and always will possess, that nothing—even time—can steal away from you. No skin care regimen or cosmetic surgeon, no matter how skilled, can make a 50-year-old look 20 again. *But it doesn't matter.* When we think of beauty, we often think in terms akin to those of the 19th-century poet Henry Wadsworth Longfellow: "How beautiful is youth! How bright it gleams." Of course, youth is magnetic and will always turn heads. But ultimately, it's serenity and confidence in yourself—the hallmarks of inner beauty—that keep heads turned, not a physically perfect yet spiritually empty face.

Thankfully, many of my patients recognize this when they tell me they actually *feel* more beautiful in their forties than they did in their twenties. Carole is 48 and has hosted an annual gathering for her women friends every December for the past 24 years. She smiled as she told me, "We've grown up together and learned to accept ourselves as we are. We used to worry about our weight, about every little thing we thought was wrong with how we looked. Now we look at each other and see real beauty—the kind of beauty that comes from inside you."

Judy, reminiscing about her 25th high school reunion, said it best. "All the women looked great. What you saw *in* their eyes was more important than the lines around their eyes."

We're all familiar with the cliché of the beautiful but insecure woman, the gorgeous creature who cannot derive any pleasure from her looks because she doesn't feel good about herself inside. (Snow White's stepmother is only one particularly self-destructive variation on this theme.) While we may not identify with this cliché, how many of us react to a compliment not by gracefully accepting it but by putting ourselves down?

Why do we do this? Are we afraid that admitting we agree makes us vain? Or is it more fundamental—do we truly not believe these compliments are earned?

Once you can locate your inner beauty and achieve a positive self-image, you will always be beautiful to yourself and to others. Honest compliments will cease to surprise you because they will merely reflect your attitude toward yourself. Instead of thinking of your outer and inner beauty as separate entities, you'll come to see them as a symbiotic continuum.

Your inner beauty enables you to take responsibility for your own happiness and to love yourself unconditionally. Once you've worked at feeling good inside and you feel secure in your own skin, you can successfully cope with the physical aspects of aging, and even have successful cosmetic surgery, if that's what you choose. By "successful," I don't mean the perfect nose or the ultimate lips. I define success as deriving enhanced feelings of beauty and self from your procedure—not because of the procedure itself but because you see the "real" you reflected back. That's what successful cosmetic surgery is all about: looking as good on the outside as you feel inside.

Beauty Reborn from the Inside Out

The rebirth of beauty in midlife has to begin on the inside, with the understanding that harmonizing inner and outer beauty can help us transcend aging. When you can embrace and truly believe the idea that transcendent beauty can be cultivated by *any* woman at *any* age, rebirth becomes possible.

You cannot change the fact that certain genes encode your facial proportions or that your facial structure will change in what our culture perceives to be a negative manner as you age. Beauty based upon bone structure and youth has the two-dimensional quality that the camera is said to "love."

What you *can* change is the way you see yourself. Transcendent beauty means looking in the mirror and never hating yourself. It's rising above a premenstrual pimple or a bad hair day, knowing that your personal charisma is what other people will see. It's feeling secure in your own, unique beauty, without the need to rate yourself against every woman you meet. And it's the courage to embrace change—even the changes of aging.

You don't have to walk into a room as if you own it, but I do want you to walk in feeling like you own *yourself*.

That's how I think of Cleopatra of ancient Egypt, unfurling herself dramatically from a carpet roll in front of an astounded Julius Caesar. Despite her flattering official portraits, it's generally accepted that she was not possessed of conventional beauty. In reality, her nose may have been long and beaky and her neck swathed in rolls of fat. Her charisma, ingenuity, and the "infinite variety" immortalized by Shakespeare made these traits irrelevant.

I'm also reminded of Anne Boleyn, the second wife of the 16th-century king, Henry VIII. She had a swarthy complexion, dark eyes, and dark hair in an era when blondness defined female beauty; she's even reputed to have had physical deformities. But she was resourceful enough to turn these to her advantage by making high-necked, long-sleeved dresses—said to be designed to conceal disfiguring moles and an extra finger—the height of fashion. She captivated the most powerful man in the nation with her magnetism and, perhaps inevitably, unnerved his subjects so much that many thought her—and eventually condemned her as—a witch.

There are modern-day transcendent beauties too, like Jill Scott, the talented young poet and R&B singer, who defines her own brand of beauty, unfettered by conventional ideas of how her hair, face, and body "should" be. History is filled with real women whose facial features are less than perfect but who are sublimely alluring because their passion for life captures our imaginations in person. My waiting room is filled with them too.

Take Zoe, for instance. She's a saleswoman in her mid-forties, blessed with a dazzling smile and extravagantly lashed eyes that sparkle with the joy of life. She's not conventionally beautiful. But she projects an aura of attractiveness, and it's easy to imagine her in her modeling days a couple of decades ago. Ask her how she keeps her verve, and she'll laugh and tell you, "It's tennis—all tennis!"

Zoe always enters my office well-informed about the procedures she's considering. She does her research and then comes to me with all her burning questions methodically entered in her pocket notebook. I may have fixed Zoe's frown lines with Botox and her smile lines with injections of fat, but it's the light within her that makes her truly content. As she says herself, "We're a great team, Doc—I work on the inside, and you help me with the outside!"

You don't have to follow a formula to be as beautiful as you can be. After all, this is not "The Rules" of beauty. The most important thing will always be to know yourself. But I'm not going to sit here and tell you that you can be supremely confident in your own, unique style of beauty without working at it at all. With a little bit of effort, every woman can be a Zoe—or a Jill Scott or a Susan Sarandon or a Barbra Streisand or a Katie Couric, or whichever contemporary beauty speaks to your soul. Together, we can work on the positive attitude, increased self-esteem, and a beauty-enhancing lifestyle. And then you may want a little outside help from your makeup, your hairstyle, and perhaps cosmetic surgery. The right mix of these elements will give you true, charismatic beauty.

True beauty is not a passive state of being, on view like Snow White in her glass box. It's not conferred on you by others, be they admirers or even cosmetic surgeons. True beauty is an active state that every woman defines, embodies, and expresses in her own fashion. In the end, your beauty is not in the eye of the beholder but in your *own* eye, an eye you have to learn to trust before you make major decisions.

The Five Red Lights of Beauty

To Kay, a personal trainer in her late forties, the formula for successful cosmetic surgery was simple.

"Obviously, the better my results, the happier I'll feel," she told me emphatically.

Unfortunately, reality is rather more complicated. And if you're interested in cosmetic surgery, or any kind of extensive facial treatment, it's vital that you realize this before you start looking for a doctor or even thinking about what you might like to improve. I don't want to downplay the importance of your finding the most skilled surgeon and of his performing his best work. But I want you to understand that you still won't be happy unless you chose to see a physician for the correct reasons. Your mindset is every bit as important as your results in determining your outcome—that is, how happy you are afterward.

I was able to explain this to Kay with an analogy drawn from her own profession.

"You're a great trainer. But suppose you had a client who was not in the right frame of mind when she began your program. Suppose she'd been pushed against her will into working out, or she had a distorted body image, or she thought losing a few inches off her hips would help her win friends. Do you think she'd be happy even if you got her in the best shape she could be?"

This same rationale underscores what I call "the red lights of beauty"—the five warning signs which practically guarantee you won't be happy if you have cosmetic surgery. If any of these five caveats applies to you, I urge you to put the brakes on any plans you have for extensive cosmetic surgery. You need to do the requisite inside work first; otherwise you may find yourself headed for disappointment at best . . . and disaster at worst.

Red Light #1. Don't Dismiss Your Motives

I believe there are "good" and "bad" reasons to have cosmetic surgery, but I don't mean "good" and "bad" from some moralistic point of view. I'm speaking from a pragmatic, experience-based perspective of which motivations lead women to happy endings, and which don't.

Many women find it difficult to simply accept the fact that looking better can make them feel better, if they're reasonable about their goals. They think that they can only fulfill their inner beauty by downplaying the importance of outer beauty. This mistaken belief that outer and inner beauty sit at opposite ends of a seesaw can keep you endlessly conflicted, especially if you're considering cosmetic surgery.

If you are secure in your inner beauty and develop it as an integral part of your beauty strategy, that actually makes you a *better* candidate for cosmetic surgery. Why? Many reasons. Because you can intuit if and when you are truly ready for it. Because you won't feel guilty about wanting to turn back the clock and look your best at any age. Because you'll understand that just as feeling good makes you look good, looking good makes you feel good.

Joy had a double impetus for visiting me: her 40th birthday and her upcoming wedding. Her beauty strategy was as methodical as her organization at the university where she taught. She made her first appointment with me a full year before her wedding, just after she'd announced her engagement. For me, it was a refreshing change from the brides-to-be who land in my office 3 weeks before their nuptials, wanting their faces to be clear in time for the big day.

Joy was basically happy with her appearance, but she had no hangups about pointing out what she didn't like. As she put it, "My face has dropped when my spirits haven't." She would be wearing her auburn hair up for the church ceremony. This would emphasize the acne scars on her cheeks and her slightly sagging jawline, both of which had become more noticeable as her skin had become less taut. And her scoopneck wedding gown would reveal the prominent sunspots and spider veins that had appeared on her chest and back after a beach vacation 5 years before.

These problems were easy for me to fix, particularly because we had plenty of time. Chemical peeling and the CoolTouch laser faded Joy's acne scars and tightened her jawline. And the Diolite laser took care of her spider veins and sunspots. Joy had no conflicts about dealing with these issues, even though her mother apparently did and criticized her for her "vanity."

"She doesn't understand," Joy told me matter-of-factly. "I'm not doing this for anyone else; it's for me. What's wrong with wanting to be the best you can be?"

To Joy, optimizing her beauty was a simple extension of her drive to pursue excellence in every aspect of her life, whether personal or professional. She was up-front about the fact that how she looked mattered to her—and she didn't need to cloak her wish to look better in order to feel comfortable fulfilling it.

Red Light #2. Make Friends with Your Self . . . Then with Your Face

Never assume that looking better will automatically cure your unhappiness. It won't, as Marie learned the hard way.

Marie had been plagued with severe acne since her early teens. Her anguish over her condition had made her stay home on prom night and avoid dating in college. She was in her early thirties when I first met her. I got her acne under control with aggressive antibiotic treatment, but the preceding years had already left a tragic signature on her face in the form of deep pitted scars. These became more noticeable as Marie progressed into her mid-thirties and her skin began to lose its elasticity. As I got to know her, I could see her already battered self-esteem slipping further, so I encouraged her to see a psychiatrist. He diagnosed her with clinical depression, and prescribed medication that helped to some extent.

Still, Marie continued to grieve over her ruined skin. She asked me several times to "get rid of all this junk on my face." It became clear to me that Marie's true objective could not be fulfilled, even by the most skilled cosmetic surgery. I could certainly improve her skin significantly, but I couldn't give her what she wanted: to travel back to time in her youth, before she had become "the girl with bad skin."

I was glad that she agreed to continue psychiatric counseling and antidepressant therapy, and I told her we should continue to discuss her treatment options. My goal was to get her to develop more realistic aims, rather than embark upon cosmetic surgery at that point. Marie continued to see me for acne treatment but soon informed me that she'd scheduled laser resurfacing with another physician who had promised to remove all her scars.

Sadly, the outcome was all too predictable. Marie had her surgery. And 2 months later, she was in tears in my office, complaining that the scars were no better than before. In fact, they were improved to some extent, but no surgery could have given Marie what she wanted. Her cosmetic surgery should never have been performed—because her inner wounds needed tending to first.

Can cosmetic surgery ever help a woman's psychological pain? I believe it can, provided that she's working on the healing through other means too. What's inside, although injured, needs to remain strong and active. Cosmetic surgery may help to heal your inner Self, but it can't give it the kiss of life.

Lorraine is a good example of how external change can mirror internal healing. She came to see me shortly after she had decided to end her marriage. Her husband of 7 years had decided to start nightclubbing again—without her. Lorraine was left literally holding the babies every evening.

Thanks to our combined efforts, Lorraine now looks somewhat younger than the 40-something mother of two that she is. What's more important is that she now looks her personal best. She never fell into the trap of blaming herself unjustly for the events in her life. Her facial makeover inspired her to adopt a macrobiotic diet and begin seriously working out. Now she is trim, fit, toned, and "ready to enter the fray," as she puts it.

Red Light #3. Don't Let the "New You" Obliterate the Inner You

"So, am I going to be a new me?" Dawn asked me with a grin as I carefully injected her forehead with Botox.

I paused for a moment and smiled back. "No, Dawn, you'll be the old you, only without frown lines."

The "new you" has become a catch word of cosmetic surgery. Like me, you're probably assailed with it every time you run across an ad from the beauty industry. We need to step back from the rhetoric and examine what that phrase really means.

I spoke before of twice-born beauty—the rebirth of your beauty when you reunite its inner and outer aspects. And of how cosmetic surgery can be a part of this process if it lets you balance what's outside with what's inside. But this transformation isn't producing a new you; it's rebirthing a *renewed* you. This isn't a mere semantic distinction. When you're renewed, you're reclaiming what you had before—the radiant, holistic beauty of your childhood. You're recognizing and including your inner Self in your renewed beauty.

To me, the promise of a "new you" is something else. This "in with the new, out with the old" philosophy implies that the old you is somehow not good enough, that the old you should be discarded and re-placed with something of your surgeon's creation. What a dangerous trap to fall into! Ads that make use of this desire for self-obliteration are specif-ically aimed—whether their creators consciously realize it or not—at women with low self-esteem.

The "new you" ideology totally fails to acknowledge the importance of your inner Self in your beauty. The "new you" transformation is brought about solely on the surface—it's what you see in the mirror, not what you see in your eyes. When you discard the old you, you're throwing it out lock, stock, and barrel, including what's inside.

Furthermore, I think we mystify cosmetic surgery enough as it is. Have you heard the fanciful reports about the face of movie star Catherine Deneuve, that it seems ageless because it's held together with pure gold stitches? The idea that cosmetic surgery metamorphoses you into a different person only increases the shroud of magical mystique. An air of mystery may be fascinating and alluring—and a great selling point—but it doesn't encourage reasoned thinking. Careful thought and objective reasoning are what you need more than anything else, if you don't want to become a victim of bad decisions.

Red Light #4. Don't Get Stage-Mothered

Never have cosmetic surgery to please someone else—like your partner or girlfriend—who's trying to push you into it. Doing so will only entrench you deeper in objectified victimhood. If your partner comments negatively about your frown lines, don't assume that fixing them will make him fall in love with you all over again. He'll probably just find something else to kvetch about. Take it from me; if he's pressuring you to have work done, the fact that you're aging is not the true problem in your relationship.

I've met many patients over the years who've told me that they "have" to fix their wrinkles or clear their acne or get rid of their double chins because somebody else was telling them to do so. And sometimes that somebody else is right there in the waiting room, telling me what I "have" to do too.

Juhi's appointment with me was made by her older sister-in-law, Rupal, who informed me on the telephone that "all her acne scars have to be gone by next month." In fact, Rupal had extensive acne scarring herself, and she'd come to see me 1 week previously. I'd had to tell her that there was not a whole lot that could be done for her type of scarring, other than surgically removing each scar individually from her face—a lengthy and painstaking procedure that would leave her with far from perfect results. I didn't think Rupal would be happy with anything less than perfection.

Now Rupal was back with Juhi. The two women presented an interesting tableau in the exam room. There was Juhi, eyes downcast, murmuring replies to my questions. And there was her sister-in-law, talking over her. When I asked Juhi if she had any acne on her back or chest, she began to shake her head. Immediately, Rupal leaped to her feet and vigorously lifted Juhi's shirt, to reveal that she did indeed have some acne on her back.

Welcome to the stage mother syndrome. Rupal couldn't get what she wanted—scar-free skin—so she was trying to live her dream through Juhi and, in doing so, assert some control over her own life. If you allow yourself to be stage-mothered into cosmetic surgery, you're pretty much doomed to failure, not only in your own eyes but in the eyes of your stage mother, who is seeking the impossible: perfection.

Sometimes the stage mother really *is* one. Twenty-year-old Cindy came to see me with her mother in tow. "Cindy's going to be an actress," her mother announced. "She needs to have her cheeks and chin liposuctioned."

Cindy didn't look like she wanted to be an actress. She didn't even look like she wanted to be in my office. And, as a rule, I don't perform liposuction on anyone who's under 25. In your teens and early twenties, your body is still finding its metabolic set point. Think back to those days, and you may well remember your weight's fluctuating by several pounds one way or another for no apparent reason. That's not the time for liposuction. The best candidate is a woman over 25 whose weight is stable (within 30 pounds of her medically defined ideal) and who has problem areas—often inherited—that persist despite her eating right and working out.

Always remember, the question you should be asking yourself is "Why am I here?" (Your doctor should also be very interested in the answer to this question.) If you don't have a good answer to that question, or if somebody else is putting answers in your mouth, you may find yourself embarking on a financially and emotionally costly voyage that leads nowhere.

Red Light #5. Don't Be Dishonest with Yourself or Your Doctor

The opposite of the stage mother syndrome is a woman's inability to admit—either to herself or to me—that she wants cosmetic surgery. She has to attribute her desires to somebody else in her life.

This situation reminds me of a charming poem by A. A. Milne, the creator of Winnie-the-Pooh. In "Binker," he writes in the voice of a little boy talking about his imaginary friend:

> *Binker isn't greedy, but he does like things to eat,*
> *So I have to say to people when they're giving me a sweet,*
> *"Oh, Binker wants a chocolate, so could you give me two?"*
> *And then I eat it for him, 'cos his teeth are rather new.*

I've met several patients in my office whose modi operandi were similar to Binker. Hilary was one of them. An energetic 43-year-old, she insisted that it was her husband—not she—who wanted her to have liposuction of her double chin and laser resurfacing of her facial wrinkles and discolorations. Somehow, her story didn't ring true. Hilary didn't seem like the kind of woman who'd let herself be stage-mothered into anything.

Plus, she was in a rush to have her procedures. She phoned me three times during the week after we first met to ask how soon she could get everything done. Was her husband pressuring her to make these calls too? I told her on the phone what I'd told her in the office—that I felt she needed time to consider her options and objectives. I was particularly concerned that her expectations were unrealistic—that she thought the surgery would leave her skin and jawline flawless. She also mentioned her money worries more than once—the expense of caring for a new baby while she and her husband were starting a new business together. The last thing I wanted was for her to dive into surgery that would squeeze her financially and then leave her disappointed.

To settle my concerns, I suggested that she come back with her husband to talk to me. As they sat in my office together, Hilary wore a bright red suit and perched on the edge of her chair. Her husband, more casually dressed, sat back, cradling their 9-month-old daughter in his arms.

"Tom's 8 years younger, and I'm only doing this for him," Hilary declared, smiling fondly at him.

"You look fine to me as you are," Tom replied, stroking the baby's head.

Hilary threw her hands in the air. "But honey, I'll look so much better. We have a *baby*. Do you want me to look like her grandmother?"

You may be able to palm off your desire for cosmetic surgery onto others, but you cannot ultimately palm off the surgery itself or its emotional aftermath. Before you can think seriously about cosmetic surgery, you must feel comfortable saying, "*I* am the one seeking this change." You must admit that in order to take emotional responsibility for your surgery. If you fail to take this responsibility, you'll never be fully satisfied with your results, no matter how good they are. You're even at a higher risk of suboptimal results, because chances are you won't be engaged sufficiently in the whole process of finding the right doctor and the right procedure.

part two

Surfacing Your Inner Beauty

chapter four

Conquering the "Ordeal by Mirror"

Nothing in life is to be feared. It is only to be understood.

—Marie Curie

Medieval witch trials often involved an Ordeal where the suspect was thrown into deep water. If you sank, you were innocent; if you floated, you were guilty of witchcraft. The innocent usually drowned. The guilty were burned at the stake.

Today a woman in midlife finds herself in a similar no-win situation, what I call the Ordeal by Mirror. If you look in a mirror and actually feel good about what you see, you're guilty of vanity. More likely, you look in the mirror and see the media-driven ideal of youthful, objectified beauty staring back mockingly over your shoulder—an ideal that can never be achieved in reality because it's airbrushed, artfully lit, and computer-enhanced. The verdict is in: you're guilty of being human; worse yet, an aging human; and, worst of all, an aging *woman*!

The first step in understanding the powerful control that mirrors have over our self-image is to appreciate their history and our love-hate relationship with them. Then you can transform the Ordeal by

Mirror into a saner, more balanced, and more joyful view of your own beauty.

The Looking Glass through Time

Our relationship with mirrors has always been tempestuous. In every culture, we've accorded them a significance that by far overshadows their utilitarian function. The special place we reserve for them in our lives is apparent in the fact that the word for "mirror" in many languages, including our own, has its roots in the Latin word for "wonder."

Mirrors were such prized possessions in ancient China that they were often buried with their owners or passed along to heirs, where it was believed that they attracted the water of life. In Egypt, they were used as amulets, and were believed to be associated with the gods, life, energy, and the divine waters of the Nile.

But mirrors date back long before this to when our ancestors first saw their reflections in water, a natural mirror. No doubt this was a fascinating experience. The terror that this could also engender is apparent in the ancient belief that catching sight of your reflection, or dreaming of it, was an omen of your impending death.

These reflections were believed to magically reveal glimpses of our fates, convey divine messages to us, and all too often ensnare us and punish us for our moral imperfections. Think of Narcissus of Greek mythology, leaning on the edge of a dark pool, bewitched—and doomed—by his love for his own exquisite reflection. Narcissus reaps the ultimate punishment for vanity, and the mirror is the instrument of his demise.

Mirrors engender such awe and fear in us that they are the focus of innumerable superstitions. Break a mirror and you've shattered your own future or, at least, condemned yourself to 7 years of bad luck. If a mirror falls and breaks by itself, watch out for imminent death in the house. The 19th-century poet Alfred, Lord Tennyson, immortalized the broken mirror as the epitome of bad luck when he wrote of the Lady of Shallot, who dies of unrequited love for the knight Lancelot:

> *The mirror crack'd from side to side;*
> *"The curse is come upon me," cried*
> *The Lady of Shalott.*

But we've often seen mirrors as positive, spiritual metaphors too. In Judaism, the mirror is a symbol for the essence of the original. And in Hinduism, your reflection represents the consciousness that is derived from your soul. Feng shui, the Chinese art of object placement to create spiritual harmony within a space, advocates the use of mirrors to redirect energy. The connection we perceive between the working of a mirror and the working of the mind is shown by our use of the word "reflect" to signify both.

Portenders of doom, instruments of fate, mesmeric objects of spiritual and sensual inspiration, mirrors arouse complex and opposing emotions. But that should not be surprising. After all, mirrors and beauty have been inextricably linked throughout human history. So it's only to be expected that our feelings about mirrors parallel—and are as conflicted as—what we feel for beauty.

Mirror, Mirror, Drive Us *off* the Wall

Our conflict over mirrors is nowhere more powerfully expressed than in the story of Snow White. The magical talking mirror brings immense pleasure over the years to its owner, Snow White's stepmother queen, by reassuring her that she is beautiful above all others. But, finally, it is the mirror that proves to be the queen's downfall. It punishes her for her vanity and evil by driving her insane with jealousy for Snow White, whose beauty has surpassed her own.

The queen's relationship-gone-bad with her mirror is an eloquent metaphor for the dilemma facing many women today. As children, we enjoy a joyful and uncomplicated relationship with mirrors. Later, this bond starts to unravel with the curse of self-consciousness. How others perceive us drowns out the sweet music of how we perceive ourselves and, in doing so, banishes the pure pleasure of a child reveling in her own image.

This curse crowds our lives with mirrors, and not just those that hang on our walls. The modern mirrors of the media—magazine covers, movies, models in the ads—bombard us on a daily basis. They all reinforce a rigid beauty "norm," an ironic term considering just how few of us are normal in this respect! And they lace the simple act of looking in the mirror with a cocktail of complex emotions: anticipation and apprehension, the hope of fantasy and the fear of reality.

Dominating it all is the feeling of inadequacy if we're not "classically" beautiful or if we have acne, scars, dark circles under our eyes—anything that doesn't exist in the land of the almighty airbrush. And it only gets worse in midlife as our first wrinkles appear. At some point—increasingly often as she gets older—every woman looks in the mirror and dislikes what she sees.

Maybe it's the frown lines you just became aware of because somebody asked you why you were angry when you weren't. Or the sunspots you know were not there a month ago. Perhaps the biggest failing of the mirror is that it doesn't reflect the wealth of wisdom and self-confidence you've accrued along your life's journey.

The most distressing part of the aging process for many women is that their faces no longer project the true image of how they feel inside. There's a mismatch between your inner self and outer persona. When what's externally on show no longer evokes a positive reaction from yourself or others, this inevitably has a negative effect on how you feel inside. My patient Lisa told me: "I used to think bad hair days were terrible enough; now I have bad face days!"

At its most graphic extreme, the Ordeal by Mirror causes physical damage. Ruby had a medical reason for taking the Ordeal by Mirror to the extreme. She inflicted deep wounds on her own face by clawing at insignificant blemishes and ended up with disfiguring scars. When she first came to see me, she had gouged out a quarter-size hole in her chin in an attempt to remove a blackhead. Fortunately, I was able to persuade her to see a psychiatrist, who prescribed therapy for obsessive-compulsive behavior. Ruby no longer destroys her face, and I was able to improve her scars with chemical peeling and laser treatments.

For many women in midlife, the wounds of self-criticism and the resultant scarring to the psyche can be just as traumatic as actual physical scars. We may judge ourselves guilty of aging—and also guilty of wanting to do something about it—day after day.

My office is full of mirrors. One of the first things I usually do when I meet a patient is to hand her a mirror so that she and I can both see what she's talking about. The reactions of my patients speak volumes about the all-pervasive effects of the Ordeal by Mirror. Jill, for instance, refuses to take the mirror at all. Carolina takes it but declares, "Do I really have to look in *that*?" Mary rests it facedown in her lap, with both hands on top of it as if to subdue it. Rina looks in the mirror briefly, then thrusts it back at me, exclaiming, "Oh, my God, the light in here is *terrible*."

And it's true, the fluorescent lighting in my office *is* harsh—but intentionally so. I need to see every imperfection in your face because that's what I'm here to fix. But *you* don't. What you need is to feel good—and confident—about yourself when you look in your mirror. Try this: close your eyes and think of someone whom you find attractive. Inevitably, your image will be of that person at her happiest and most confident. That's because feeling good about yourself really *does* make you look good.

Feeling comfortable about your appearance is a prerequisite to freeing yourself from the opinions of others—society, partners, friends, whomever—and becoming secure in your own, unique beauty. The challenge is to commit to breaking the habits of a lifetime so you can escape the Ordeal by Mirror.

Your Reflection Is Nothing Personal

How can you handle all those faces in all those mirrors and make sense of—and peace with—their belittling voices? The feminist fallacy tells you to do this by blaming modern society in general, and modern men in particular, for valuing beauty. But blaming society only perpetuates the knee-jerk denial of one incontrovertible fact: it's as natural for us to appreciate human beauty as it is for us to swoon over a gorgeous bed of roses, a designer home, or a wonderful painting.

I think the real key to overcoming the Ordeal by Mirror is for us all—beholders and beheld—not to take the issue of beauty so *personally*. If we can enjoy the sublime artifice of a filter-enhanced sunset in a movie without feeling angry that sundown viewed from our own backyards does not match up, why can we not accept the image of idealized beauty the media throw at us as a mere fantasy, not something we have to fruitlessly quest for in ourselves or demand in others?

Think of the Taj Mahal, the famed mausoleum built by an Indian emperor as an eternal tribute to the beloved wife he lost. In the picture postcards, it's a breathtaking marble edifice set amid stately gardens with crystal waters. See it in person and it's still beautiful, but there's imperfection too: the missing precious stones have been pried out of the chipped and crumbling walls by invaders and robbers; packs of howling dogs prowl nightly; the ever-present peddlers hawk plastic key chains. When you stand on the site itself, you understand why all the pictures are taken front-on—because this obscures the industrial smokestacks that are so visible from other viewpoints.

Like a magazine model, the Taj Mahal is always photographically captured from its best angle to preserve the illusion of perfect beauty. Yet the Taj Mahal of our reality and the one of the media can coexist harmoniously in our minds without our having to invoke a societal conspiracy to explain their differences.

It's vitally important for us as women to understand and to make peace with this, both for ourselves and for our children. The mirrors on the wall and the mirrors of the media will always be there; they tap into our innate love of idealized beauty and they sell too many jars of cream, cars, clothes, and movies to ever go away. We can't spend a lifetime pretending they don't exist. And we can't raise our children in a mirror-free world.

Our Daughters' Beauty, Our Own

Recently Naomi, who's 18, was in my office, having laser hair removal, while her mother thumbed through *YM* magazine in the waiting room. She paused at the back cover to scrutinize a photograph of a young woman with impossibly perfect skin and a computer-elongated body and asked me what I thought of it.

"Well, it's a nice picture; the lighting's very good," I ventured.

"Yes, but look at it," Naomi's mother replied. "What are we teaching our daughters by exposing them to *this*?"

Although I chose not to answer her at that moment—experience had told me she would not be open to my thoughts on this subject—my answer is that we can teach our daughters anything we choose to teach them. I think one of the most important lessons they can learn is that they *can* appreciate the fantasy beauty of fairy tales—Snow White skin and all—without feeling inadequate about the imperfections that make *them* real and human. After all, that's part of what growing up is all about: learning to distinguish fantasy from reality.

When my own daughter was in second grade, she came home in some anguish one day because a thoughtless classmate had commented about the hair on her upper lip. I didn't regale her with stories of the Taj Mahal, but I did point out that even a perfect-looking cover girl has blemishes—a revelation that shocked her. She was surprised to learn that I was also troubled by my "excess" hair as a child and adolescent—all the more so because my own mother was unusually hair-free for an Indian woman and I'd never examined another Indian girl at close quarters. By the time we finished our conversation, her newfound knowledge of what airbrushing can do, the myriad of methods for removing hair, and other fascinating topics had wiped all thoughts of inadequacy from her mind. Her animated face was proof positive that knowledge is power.

You can also look at a magazine cover and see it not as an affront to your own "imperfect" appearance but as what it truly is: an icon of objectified beauty that can hurt you only if you let it. You can even allow yourself to appreciate this icon as art in its own way, without relating it directly to yourself. In doing so, you empower yourself to develop your subjective beauty to its fullest, unimpeded and unthreatened by objective beauty—or by others who would hold you to its impossible standards.

See Yourself With Love—
and Love What You See

A vital step in appreciating your own beauty is to harness the positive power of your mirror image. Keep in mind that, when you look in the mirror, you never *truly* see yourself as others see you. While it is your mirror image that you carry with you throughout your day and life, your mirror image is not simply a copy of your true self. A mirror actually reverses you. Why does this matter? Because, in reversing you, a mirror reverses your asymmetries—the mismatches between your right and left sides. And we *all* have them. Whether it's one eye that's differently shaped, one side of your mouth that's a little fuller than the other, one eyebrow that arches more than its companion, there's not a woman (or man) in the world whose face is identical on the right and left.

This reversal is the reason we find projections of ourselves as we actually are—and as others see us—less attractive than projections of our mirror image. It's the reason you may not enjoy looking at photographs of yourself: You're seeing the reverse of what you see in the mirror—for example, that more arched eyebrow is on the left instead of the right—and this can lend the photograph an alien quality.

From the ancient Greeks to Leonardo da Vinci in his book *The Proportions of Man* to today's depictions of perfectly proportioned supermodels, we've been preoccupied for millennia with facial and bodily symmetry as a necessity for ideal beauty. And with good reason—in our species, as in all others, symmetry of right and left sides is an indicator of good health and freedom from inherited or acquired disease that could cause uneven or stunted development. That's why animals tend to choose symmetrical mates and why bees prefer to pollinate symmetrical flowers. What's more, left-to-right symmetry is also a hallmark of youth. One of the cardinal signs of aging is that your face starts to become less symmetrical.

But there's more to the symmetry story than meets the eye. It's certainly true that we perceive more beauty in a face whose right and left sides match than in one whose sides don't. However, some investigators have suggested that certain types of asymmetry may actually make a face *more* attractive because a perfectly symmetrical face can appear emotionless and unnaturally masklike. That's why the quest for perfect beauty is ultimately pointless.

There's another important way in which your mirror image differs from the image that others see. If you're like most women, you probably keep your face relatively immobile when you look in the mirror. Thus, your mirror image is static and bears little trace of the dynamic vibrancy which reflects your underlying personality. The mirror transforms you into a stagnant reflection whose physical irregularities stand out in sharp relief, because they are stripped bare of the softening, real-life animation that others see when they look at your face.

Your reflection in the mirror is imperfect because it doesn't show you how you truly look to others. But it's the only image of yourself that you possess. The challenge is to transform that mirror image from emotional baggage into emotional support. I suggest three ways of doing this.

1. See the whole picture. This means throwing away your magnifying mirror. Keep it for inserting your contact lenses if you must, but don't use it for self-appraisal or even to apply makeup. Now, you may retort that you need your magnifying mirror to tweeze your eyebrows. But I hope you'll make it obsolete for this purpose too, once I've explained why you shouldn't be shaping your own eyebrows anyway!

Human skin was not intended to be examined in microdetail. When you do so, you only inflict torture upon yourself. Many of the blemishes that are all too evident in your magnifying mirror are hardly visible, if at all, to the human eye—particularly to an eye other than yours. The danger of overexamining your skin is that you become focused on insignificant imperfections—and asymmetries—that prevent you from feeling beautiful. Remember that even the most beautiful painting looks like an unruly mess of brushstrokes when viewed too closely.

2. See yourself in the best possible light. More pragmatic advice: do whatever it takes to feel good about looking in your mirror. Backlight or soft-light it, avoid unflattering fluorescent lamps, make its reflection something you like. The type of lighting I want you to avoid is what you find in a typical hotel bathroom. You know what I mean—that harsh fluorescent glare that makes everyone's skin look sickly and every imperfection stand out in sharp relief.

You can really have fun experimenting with different types and directions of lighting and will be amazed at the difference it makes to your face. I want you to go through your day with a positive image of your own appearance. You can do this only if you quite literally see yourself in the best possible light from the moment you wake up. Take the time to find the right mirror and the right light for your face.

My patient Evelyn recently showed me a photo of her bedroom, which she'd just finished redecorating. What struck me the most was her mirror, which she'd found in a consignment store specializing in antiques. It was actually three mirrors resting within a hinged filigree silver frame atop her dressing table.

"What a great mirror!" I exclaimed, and Evelyn laughed.

"Yes, I fell in love with it as soon as I saw it. The frame is so gorgeous it makes whatever you see in it look great too. And I can adjust the angles of the hinges however I like, so I can have whatever mirror face I want!"

3. Look at yourself through different eyes. To paraphrase the Scottish poet Robert Burns: "We should have the gift of seeing ourselves as others see us." I have a patient, Cathy, who used to be preoccupied with the size of her pores. Even after I'd improved her skin significantly with at-home treatments and in-office salt macrodermabrasion, she reported that her magnifying mirror still told the same depressing story. Finally, I advised her, "Go ask your closest girlfriend what she thinks of your skin." To Cathy's amazement—but not mine—the friend saw only a 50-year-old with glorious skin. This realization was the turning point for Cathy, who is now free of her insecurities—and of her magnifying mirror.

The lesson is that we're the least objective observers of our own beauty. I've asked you to define beauty on your own terms, not others'. To do this, you need to become more appreciative and forgiving of yourself. That doesn't mean glossing over or ignoring what distresses you, but it does mean being an equal-opportunity beholder, seeing and valuing your own good points just as you see and value them in others.

chapter five

The Seven Emotions That Age Us

The most wasted of all days is one during which you did not laugh.

—Sebastian Roch Nicholas Chamfort

*M*y first thought when Yvette walked into my office was "Did *I* do that?"

I'd treated Yvette's frown lines and crow's-feet with Botox the week before, and everything had gone well. Or, at least, so I'd thought. But here she was, back for her follow-up appointment, with a huge black eye!

"So . . . how's the Botox?" I inquired casually.

"Oh, fine," Yvette replied.

I knew instantly something was wrong. Yvette—a 40-something homemaker and longtime patient—was usually chatty and cheerful. The monosyllabic response and her lack of eye contact were totally uncharacteristic. Still, her usual vivaciousness belied the fact that she was going through an acrimonious divorce. Her soon-to-be ex-husband was a high-profile attorney who was not afraid to use his professional connections to get what he wanted personally.

"And . . . the bruise, how did that happen?" I continued.

Her reply made me almost wish that my Botox injections *were* the culprit.

"Well, Philip and I had a little altercation. He came to the house very late and very drunk, and he was screaming and threatening me, so I locked him out. But he kicked in the back door and decided to knock me down and punch me in the face."

She looked up at me for the first time and continued. "It's okay—I went to the police station and had photos taken. And I've asked for a restraining order. I mean, there's no doubt who the aggressor was—he weighs about 100 pounds more than I do."

Incredible as it might seem, Yvette was actually perking up before my eyes as she told her story. "It's okay," she repeated reassuringly. "Life goes on. I worked out for an hour at the gym this morning, and I'm going to my painting class after I see you. The bruise is outside, not inside."

Yvette's words still echo in my mind. I was amazed by her resilience, and it made me realize that while we all get bruised by life—though not necessarily in such an extreme manner and hopefully not physically—we always have the control over how we deal with these slings and arrows.

While treating my patients over the years, I've watched many women learn to heal themselves after enduring painful situations. I've also watched others flounder, seemingly unable to grow beyond the pain. In my experience, the women who struggle the most tend to be ruled by at least one of seven emotions: envy, fear, guilt, anger, self-criticism, pessimism, and perfectionism.

These seven negative emotions bruise our souls and, in doing so, age us and make us small. If you let these negative feelings control your life, they will destroy your beauty by dwarfing your inner spirit. If you can redirect the energy you're expending on these emotions into positive thoughts and actions, your spirit will soar and you can express the highest part of your self. Then you can not only value your beauty but also celebrate it.

The key to defusing these negative emotions is to demystify them. And you can do this only by understanding why they are so visceral and how they relate specifically to the beauty chase.

Envy

Oh, how bitter a thing it is to look into happiness through another man's eyes.

—William Shakespeare

Of all the negative emotions we can express, envy is the one that unsettles us the most. We can excuse other negative emotions, such as anger or guilt, as misguided but well-intentioned; but envy is so completely unbecoming that it is indefensible. There's no way to sugarcoat envy, which is probably why we resort to euphemisms, like "the green-eyed monster," to describe it.

Envy strikes a chord particularly where women and beauty are concerned because it conjures up the image of an aging, resentful crone, the mainstay of our fairy tales. Think of Snow White's stepmother queen, Rapunzel's witch, or Sleeping Beauty's wicked fairy.

Envy is the emotion most destructive for your beauty strategy because it not only wastes your energy; it also misdirects you. If you spend your time hating and feeling bitter about another woman's perceived excellence, you'll be blinded to your own good points. If you don't appreciate your own unique set of attributes, this prevents you from accepting that you can ever achieve excellence yourself.

When Kristin came to see me, her chief complaint was the texture of her skin. "I've had oily skin and open pores since I was a kid," she told me. "I don't know why I had to inherit my father's skin and not my mother's. Hers is perfect, even now that she's in her sixties. She has no pores on her face at all."

Kristin had indeed inherited her Italian father's skin. But instead of seeing its positive points—its lustrous olive tone and resistance to wrinkling—she saw only the negatives when she looked in the mirror. Conversely, she saw only the positives in her mother's Scandinavian skin without seeing the other side of the coin: the fact that her mother's skin was more prone to spider veins and wrinkles.

The turnaround began for Kristin when I put her on a regimen of alternating salt macrodermabrasion treatments and facials. In a few weeks, her pores looked less prominent and her excess shine was gone. She was then able to view her skin—and herself—in a more rational light.

Sally resented her best friend, Madge, who was also my patient, because her eyes were "so perfect." They certainly were a lovely shade of green (and they looked even better after I'd treated Madge with Botox to smooth out her crow's-feet). But what Sally didn't know was that Madge herself was discontent because she coveted Sally's thick, wavy hair!

If your focus is only on what others have and you don't, you'll never be happy *or* beautiful. And it's not just envy of those close to us that holds us back. Marianne came in for a consultation about fat injections to enhance her lips. She brought a glamour magazine to my office, pointed at a pouty young model, and said, "Make my lips like hers." When I paused, she continued. "I've got more photos of people's lips at home, and I'll bring them with me next time so you can see what I want."

I spent most of that consultation with Marianne explaining to her that I couldn't—and wouldn't—give her somebody else's lips. What I could—and did—do was to make her own lips, which were shapely but had thinned over the years, look as good as they possibly could. And Marianne was ultimately delighted with those results.

There's another type of envy that is just as toxic . . . the envy of yourself as you used to be. Were your lips fuller and your skin tighter when you were 20? Perhaps so. But let's be honest—at that age, you were probably fixated on your premenstrual pimples, rather than reveling in your youthful beauty. You cannot feel beautiful, at any age, if you're preoccupied with the images of others and the ghosts of yesteryear. Letting go of those images is an important step on the road to transcendent beauty.

Fear

Life shrinks or expands in proportion to one's courage.

—Anaïs Nin

Are you afraid to look in the mirror and admit what you'd like to change? Afraid of change itself? Or afraid of what others will think if you change?

Fear is the wall that separates you from your desires. You must surmount it to reach your goals.

Until she came to see me, Frances had let fear control her. During our first meeting, she said, "I live in a small town, and people will crucify me if they find out I've had anything done." In light of this concern, we avoided any major procedures and opted instead for those that involved no recovery time: salt macrodermabrasion to even out her skin tone and subtly improve her wrinkles, Botox to relax her frown lines, and Diolite laser treatment to remove the spider veins on her nose. She was delighted and relieved when the only comments her neighbors made were compliments on how well-rested she looked. When her crucifixion never came to pass, she was able to see that her fear of being "found out" was really a manifestation of her own fear of change.

Change is an inevitable fact of life, and aging is perhaps the scariest of all changes. It reminds us we're mortal. By extension, this makes our efforts to reverse aging seem frightening too. Sometimes one small change has the power to transform your life. This can certainly be a terrifying prospect, both to you and those around you. But, remember that change is the only way we evolve and grow.

Mira was afflicted with a rare skin condition called morphea, which had caused one side of her face to become sunken in so that she looked lopsided. Mira had lived with this condition for years. She couldn't say what had suddenly made her visit me one day in search of a cure. By the time she came to me, the disease that had destroyed one side of her face was no longer active, but its results were all too apparent.

Mira's husband was against her having any treatment, but she was utterly determined. I was able to even up Mira's face by harvesting fat from her buttock and injecting it into the sunken areas of her face. She told me that for the first time in 15-or-so years, she could look in the mirror without cringing.

What happened next was dramatic. Mira's husband became increasingly angry and verbally abusive. Meanwhile, Mira moved on from "corrective" cosmetic surgery to the purely aesthetic. By the time she was halfway through a series of chemical peels to improve the discolorations and freckles on her face, she and her husband were separated.

Had cosmetic surgery put Mira's marriage on the rocks? I don't think so. What it had done was expose the fact that the relationship was unequal; it was based on the fact that Mira was the "imperfect" one. For years, Mira had been afraid to change her appearance because it might change her relationship. When she lost her fear and her imperfection was removed, the dynamics of her marriage were shaken up, putting her on equal terms with her husband. She was no longer the imperfect one, and that made her husband angry—and afraid.

Many of my patients come to me because they want to stave off change. Maybe they want to stop time or preserve a marriage or keep a job. What they learn is that becoming more beautiful—or more youthful—is a willful transformation that's impossible if we're ruled by fear of change.

Guilt

If we are not ashamed to think it, we should not be ashamed to say it.

—Marcus Tullius Cicero

I talked earlier about why we feel guilty about pursuing beauty and staving off the signs of aging. These conflicts have polarized beauty in our minds—youth versus age, inner versus outer beauty, natural versus artificial enhancements—rather than allowed us to see the full range of options and types of beauty. As women, we're cast either in the role of Snow White, a passive object on display, or as the stepmother queen, aging and vengeful. Guilt smothers our souls and prevents us from expressing the beauty within us.

So many of my initial consultations with patients are dominated by a sense of guilt and the fear that resorting to cosmetic surgery to fight the aging process will be punished by discovery and ridicule, by a surgical disaster, or by moral retribution. But the truth is, cosmetic surgery doesn't just go wrong randomly. There's invariably a reason why. And invariably this reason was avoidable.

Take Nia, who could not lose the double chin she'd developed while pregnant with twins, despite a healthy diet and regular exercise that had helped her shed most of the excess weight she'd gained. Even before I told her so, she knew that liposuction of her chin and neck was the only remedy; the tendency to develop a double chin is hereditary and thus largely resistant to exercise or weight loss.

In Nia's case, she'd inherited her chin from her father. But she hesitated because she was afraid that "I won't be me anymore if I do something unnatural." She was scared that "maybe I'll end up deformed if I mess with how I was meant to be."

I pointed out to Nia that she'd already had other procedures, like orthodontic straightening of her teeth and eyebrow shaping, that had changed how she was "naturally." But she didn't feel guilty about them, probably because they were not directly connected to *aging*.

"Nobody, least of all me, is trying to push you into this procedure," I told her. "But your decision should be a rational one, based on facts rather than illogical emotions."

After much soul-searching, Nia decided to go ahead with the liposuction. One look at her face just a week later confirmed that she'd made the right decision. Her newly firm jawline had restored her face to its original, beautiful heart shape. But it was the light in her eyes that truly spoke volumes.

"I can't thank you enough for this," she said, smiling. "It's like I was carrying around this burden and now it's been lifted from me. I only regret I didn't do this sooner."

Guilt is at its most damaging when it causes you to make hasty and ill-considered decisions. That's what happened to Nancy, who came to see me because she had white scars around her mouth after laser resurfacing by another physician. Unfortunately, this type of scarring is extremely difficult to treat, and I had to inform Nancy that her scars would probably be permanent despite my best efforts.

"I was such a fool," she told me. "After I'd already had this done, I found out that I was only the second patient the doctor had ever treated with laser resurfacing."

Of course, the physician was to blame for failing to inform Nancy of his inexperience. He'd not only botched the procedure; one look at Nancy told me it wasn't even the correct procedure for her skin type and pattern of aging. But why had Nancy failed to ask even the most basic questions of this doctor before she'd placed herself—and her face—in his hands?

"Unlike the other doctors I'd seen before, this one didn't make me feel ashamed of wanting to do something about my wrinkles," she explained. "He was very eager to treat me."

If you feel guilty about having cosmetic surgery, you're less likely to investigate the issue thoroughly and more likely to fall into the arms of the first surgeon who accepts you and doesn't make you feel vain or frivolous. If you're secure in the knowledge that you have a right to define your own beauty, you'll have the strength to get your questions answered and to get the kind of care you deserve.

Anger

Holding on to anger is like grasping a hot coal with the intent of throwing it at someone else; you are the one getting burned.

—Buddha

Anger is an unavoidable, and sometimes appropriate, part of life. But getting angry about another woman's beauty or your own perceived lack of beauty is sheer irony because anger is the antithesis of beauty—it simply erases it. After all, it was Snow White's stepmother's rage—at her own loss of youth, at the magic mirror for noticing it, and at Snow White for supplanting her as "the fairest of them all"—that destroyed her own beauty.

We've all seen this anger in the woman who's only half joking when she says of a beautiful rival, "I hate her." Or in the resentful looks some women throw at anyone who's younger—and therefore more nubile—than they are. I see this anger increasing in many women as they approach midlife. If your concept of beauty is that it's a gift capriciously bestowed upon an undeserving few, why wouldn't you be angry with such unfairness?

Holly was an elegant and strikingly angular 45-year-old whose husband—a bodybuilder—had left her to live with a woman who was 16 years younger. Her first few visits to my office were dominated by the anger she felt, which was primarily directed at her husband's mistress, whom she called "the schoolgirl."

I'm not a professional therapist, but I could see Holly needed one, to work out her feelings of anger and betrayal, so I recommended she make an appointment. What I could do was help restore her self-esteem with a few simple procedures and an at-home skin care regimen. Along with the steps she was taking with her therapist, feeling good outside helped Holly to feel good inside. The bitter references to "the schoolgirl" stopped as Holly was able to let go of the past and focus on taking charge of her present and future.

Lily, a graphics designer in her mid-fifties, was angry at herself for her sun worship in her younger days. "There I was, covered in baby oil and iodine, roasting away," she told me. "And look at me now—I'm a total mess. I even have wrinkles on my earlobes."

It took Lily a while to understand that her anger was unfounded. After all, she'd come of age in the era when a tan was considered to be a hallmark of good health. Her own mother was forever urging her to "get some color on your face."

I was able to reverse much of Lily's premature aging with chemical peeling of her face—including her earlobes. Instead of wasting her energy on anger, she's since redirected it into sun protection. She's now one of my most sun-smart patients, and she protects her newly rejuvenated skin religiously whatever the weather. She's ingeniously found matching wraps or shawls for every short-sleeved outfit she wears while driving, has a great collection of hats for all occasions, and is a huge fan of spray-on sunscreen "because it doesn't make me feel sticky or smell like a piña colada." She even schedules her golf games in the early morning or late afternoon, when the sun's rays are less damaging.

What I want most for you is to feel secure in your own, unique brand of beauty. You can celebrate your own beauty without denigrating the beauty of others. You can value the beauty of midlife and the beauty of youth as two sides of the same coin, as long as you accept the fact that true beauty is within your reach, as it is within the reach of every woman.

Self-Criticism

Suicide is the most sincere form of self-criticism.

—Anonymous

The Ordeal by Mirror—both over-examining your face and then feeling guilty about it—is only one arena of self-criticism. Do you accept compliments gracefully, or do you feel unworthy of them? Are you self-conscious—or even incredulous—when people notice your positive attributes rather than your negative ones? Do you walk into a crowded room confidently—or preoccupied with your crow's-feet, your drooping mouth, or whatever part of yourself you love to hate?

Christine was in her late thirties, and my first impression of her was that here was a woman who simply did not feel beautiful. She walked into my office with her head hung low, her face hidden behind large glasses and even larger hair. When I asked her what her problems were, she replied, "Everything about me is wrong."

She told me that she had booked my last appointment of the day so that she wouldn't have to meet other patients in the waiting room. As I continued talking and listening to Christine, it became apparent that she knew—and hated—every imperfection on her face.

The first step I took to boost Christine's self-esteem was to clear up her acne and fade her acne scars. I did this with antibiotic pills and creams, in combination with salt macrodermabrasion sessions. I encouraged Christine to wear her hair up and to cut back on her makeup, to show off her now clear skin. She would still come in caked in makeup every once in a while, but I would always ask her to wash it all off before we even began to talk. I wanted her to feel comfortable exposing her naked face—and her naked soul—to me.

I can see that Christine still feels unworthy and inadequate at times, and that's normal—we all have those moments. But she definitely feels better about herself. I can tell by her poise and her confident stride as she enters a room, by her newly updated wardrobe, and most of all by the fact that she no longer dreads meeting others when she visits me for her appointments. When I told her the other day how beautiful she looked in green, how wonderfully it matched her eyes, she smiled shyly, blushed a little, and said, "I guess it does."

Being beautiful means being comfortable in your own skin. To realize your full beauty, you need to quiet the belittling commentary inside and give voice to positive self-esteem. The Hindu holy book, the *Bhagavad Gita* tells us, "If you want to see the brave, look at those who can forgive." The greatest bravery is to forgive *yourself*.

Pessimism

Not in the clamor of the crowded street,
Not in the shouts and plaudits of the throng,
But in ourselves, are triumph and defeat.

—Henry Wadsworth Longfellow

During our initial consultations, many of my patients express their view of the aging process as combat. They speak of "fighting" their wrinkles, and voice frustration at what they perceive as a losing battle.

The only way that you *can* win the battle is to believe that you will. Some women march into my office, their heads and expectations held high. And some, like Susan, creep in with little hope of any achievement.

Susan, an office administrator in her early forties, came to see me because her sister, Sarah, 5 years her senior, was my patient. Susan had been shocked at a recent family reunion when a distant cousin assumed that she was the older sister. Sarah noticed her distress and gave her my card.

Three months later, Susan still had not booked an appointment with me. So Sarah had called, done it for her, and escorted her to my office.

"Susan's out in the sun a lot because of her kids," Sarah told me.

Susan rolled her eyes and retorted, "Well, it's easy for you to criticize; you don't have children, so you don't have to be at all the soccer games. There's no way I can avoid the sun, so there's no point my trying to."

Both sisters had inherited the tendency to develop rosacea, characterized by the onset—often in midlife—of facial redness and easy flushing, spider veins on the nose and cheeks, and acne pimples.

Sarah, a yoga enthusiast who believed her body was a temple, was not eager to take antibiotic pills or other internal medications. But it was vitally important to her that her rosacea was controlled because she was a motivational speaker. "I can't stand up there in front of all those people looking like a tomato," she said. Diolite laser treatment had taken care of the spider veins, and Sarah's ruddy complexion was tamed by green tea serum (which also helped the wrinkles around her eyes) and antibiotic lotion.

Looking at the sisters together, I could easily see how Sarah might be mistaken for the younger of the two. But this wasn't just because she'd had cosmetic surgery and Susan hadn't. Sarah's eyes were bright with anticipation, and she radiated a vibrant love of life. Susan, on the other hand, looked down in the mouth and down at heart.

The sisters had similar skin types and patterns of rosacea, so the regimen I recommended to Susan was almost a carbon copy of the one I'd given Sarah. But her reactions to it were quite different. When I discussed stress reduction, she rolled her eyes again and declared, "Easy for you to say. I have three teenage boys at home, so how am I supposed to relax these days?" When I gave her some information about laser treatments, she invoked her family again and asked exactly how she was supposed to afford that.

"It's only a few hundred dollars, and it can be my treat," Sarah interjected quickly.

I saw Susan for follow-up 1 month later. She complained that her skin was no better. But later, during the visit, she admitted that she hadn't even filled the prescription I'd written or followed any of the three-step, 7-minute skin care routine I'd recommended.

"I just don't see the point," she told me. "I don't have the time anymore to do all this stuff at home."

Of course, Susan was time-challenged and energy-challenged— probably much more so than her free-living, single sister. More than anything, however, Susan had simply given up.

If you look in the mirror and see a worn-out shadow of your former self, then that's what you'll be. You can rise above this only if you're prepared to look beyond that mirror image and wholeheartedly see the possibilities that lie within you. To do this, you have to lose your fear of defeat. The worst failure is not defeat, but never to have tried.

Perfectionism

I think perfectionism is based on the obsessive belief that if you run carefully enough, hitting each stepping-stone just right, you won't have to die.

—Anne Lamott

The final emotion that keeps us small is the most insidious. Perfectionism defeats us on so many levels. Perfect beauty exists only in magazines and on movie screens. We are all born asymmetrical—our left and right sides don't match perfectly—and thus imperfect. Plus, we become more asymmetrical as we age. Scrutinize your or your best friend's smile or eyes and you'll see what I mean.

I meet many patients in my office who seek perfection. Their supposed flaws frustrate them and make them very unhappy. I can talk most of them out of their perfectionism by explaining the difference between the fantasy of perfect beauty and the reality of imperfect beauty. But some patients are immune to this logic.

For instance Patricia, who's 48, brought her own magnifying mirror to my office and pointed out every wrinkle and freckle she wished to be rid of. Many of them were almost imperceptible, so she had marked them with a pen to make sure that I could see them. She told me that she was so embarrassed about her skin that she didn't even like her husband to see her without makeup.

"I'm not interested in a partial fix," Patricia declared. "Whatever I have done, I want to be sure that it solves my problems completely."

Within 10 minutes of meeting Patricia, I realized that she would be unhappy with whatever procedure she had, no matter how well I or any other surgeon performed it. It was therefore in her best interest not to pursue cosmetic surgery at all. I discussed this with her, and she left my office with a cleanser, a couple of creams to use at home . . . and her magnifying mirror.

Patricia is an extreme example. But perfectionism permeates all our lives to some degree. We're societally conditioned to strive for it in every arena: the perfect relationship, the perfect job, perfect children—and the perfect face. If we turn away from perfection, we risk being viewed by others—and ourselves—as unimaginative or unambitious or just plain failures.

An important step on your path to beauty is to say no to perfectionism, regardless of what others may think. As Alexander Pope put it:

Whoever thinks a faultless piece to see
Thinks what ne'er was, nor is, nor e'er shall be.

When you wish for perfect skin, you're wishing for the impossible. A little imperfection is beautiful because it's natural. It proves you're human—and what could be more beautiful?

That's why I even out obvious asymmetry but deliberately allow for slight imperfection in many of the procedures I perform. I want my patients to look natural and for their surgery to be undetectable, if they wish. That way, their faces don't telegraph their cosmetic surgery to the world. They can always choose whether or not to tell others what they've had done.

Whatever your path to beauty, the value of slight imperfection is a vital lesson to learn. If you're chasing perfection—whether in your meditation regimen, your fitness program, your diet, or your cosmetic surgery—you're going to be disappointed, no matter how good your results.

chapter six

The Six Principles of Transcendent Beauty

We are all born for love. . . . It is the
principle of existence and its only end.

—Benjamin Disraeli

We thrive on love. Look at a child, a human being unvarnished by pretense, self-protection, or self-consciousness, and you'll see that all she really wants is to know that she is loved. Ultimately, that's all we seek when we're adults too. This desire for love inspires us, fascinates us, and makes us human. And it all begins with ourselves. There's no denying it—you can't really begin to be loved by others until you love yourself.

My six principles of transcendent beauty have one common goal: to teach you how to love yourself unconditionally and, in doing so, to develop your inner beauty. From this point of strength, you can work outward on your path to transcendent beauty. The spiritual and emotional maturity you accrue as you pass through life helps you to locate your inner beauty, to develop it, and finally to surface it in your face.

To me, transcendent beauty is the ultimate expression of love for yourself—a beauty that rises above physical limitations and endures the passage of time. It's the 30-year-old who I *know* will still be beautiful when she's 60 because there's so much more to her than good hair, smooth skin, and pretty eyes. It's the steady wisdom I see in the eyes of Rosalind, who discovered meditation when she was nearly 50, or the compassion in the smile of Martha, the ex-dancer who walks in beauty in her eighth decade. It's an allure that's out of all proportion to a woman's outside appearance, a glow from within that lights up her whole person and draws you in.

Loving yourself unconditionally doesn't mean you will go on the defensive or into denial about your faults. Instead, you will acknowledge your faults and love yourself despite them. You may find this hard to do where beauty is concerned. Many women find it challenging because they've allowed themselves to be pushed back onto the ropes of inadequacy, guilt, and shame by others and even by themselves. Evolution and society have conditioned a woman to look for approval—and by extension love—from outside sources rather than from within. Even those closest to her—particularly the men in her life—may not understand this need at all.

So often, the woman who strides confidently into the waiting room looking and acting like a million dollars becomes someone quite different when she enters the privacy zone of my exam room. Time after time, I listen to the husband or partner of one of my patients, and he raves about how unflustered by others' opinions she is, how secure in her appearance, and how unconcerned with the beauty chase. And I know that this man has never seen, and will never see, the side of this woman that I have seen. I spend a good part of every day seeing—and hearing—women at their most vulnerable. At times, their vulnerability is shocking.

Take Sheila. To the outside world, she seemed to have it all. She'd been married for more than 20 years to her high school sweetheart, with whom she shared a multi-acre horse farm in a beautiful enclave of Virginia. Sheila spent her time breeding horses and traveling to shows with her teenage daughter, Colleen, a highly-regarded competitive rider. Her son, a high school sophomore, was a straight-A student and an accomplished athlete. Several times a year, the whole family would take off for various exotic locations—the home they owned in Bermuda, their Florida villa overlooking a golf course, or a ski chalet in the Swiss Alps.

Sheila made sure I knew all this and more during our first few meetings. Initially it was hard to believe she was the busy mother of two—her impeccable outfits always showed off her slight but well-toned physique, and she turned the heads of everyone she passed in my office. Several of my staff commented on her poise and elegance. Her face was warm and vibrant, and her voice, with an endearing hint of an Irish lilt, seemed ever-ready to burst into laughter.

Sheila's been my patient for more than 5 years now. It took me a while to see what lay beneath that perfect surface. Her marriage was stormy, and what she wanted most in this world, she couldn't have: the consistent approval and love of her husband. Because of this, Sheila felt unable to love or even approve of herself.

I always knew when things were going well with her husband because the light in her eyes, visible from clear across the waiting room, would remain illuminated when she walked into the exam room to see me. When things were going badly, the light would still be on in public but quickly fade once we were alone, face-to-face.

Sheila raked in the compliments after I fixed her frown lines with Botox, enhanced her shapely but thin lips with fat and collagen injections, and chemically peeled away the facial discolorations she'd developed during her pregnancies. But to her these compliments rang hollow.

"I always feel like people are just saying it—they don't really mean it," she told me during one appointment.

I could make Sheila shine on the surface, but I couldn't make her shine within without her cooperation. She loved herself only when she felt loved. And no amount of pep talking from me or professional therapy from her sympathetic psychiatrist could change this until Sheila empowered herself to seek that change.

The trigger was when her daughter, Colleen, fell from her horse during a competition, broke her arm, and was unable to ride for several months. Suddenly without the usual hours of practice, life was empty for Colleen—and for Sheila too. Without her daily distraction, Sheila was forced to confront something she'd been evading for more than a decade by making sure she "never had the time" to deal with it: her own negative opinion of herself. This could have broken her, but instead it made her.

With the help of her therapist—and perhaps with a little help from me since I knew Sheila quite well by then and could speak to her frankly—she was able to make peace with herself. She could accept that she was not perfect and that she was in part responsible for the ups and downs in her marriage. She was finally able to see that despite her faults, she was worthy of love—from herself and from others.

The Swedish philosopher-scientist Swedenborg wrote that love in its essence is spiritual fire. Nowhere is this truer than in the way you love yourself. If you rely on others to light your fire, there may always be a day when the fire goes out. But if you appreciate the constancy of your spiritual beauty, you can love yourself wholeheartedly, unconditionally—and realistically. Follow these life principles, and you can keep the fire blazing forever.

Principle 1: You Must Feel Beautiful Before You Can Look Beautiful

As the old saying goes, "There is no cosmetic for beauty like happiness." Feeling beautiful is a prerequisite to being beautiful.

My patient Leanne is the kind of school bus driver that every mother would want for her child. She exudes a positivity that touches everyone who meets her, even my other patients who sit with her for just a few minutes in my waiting room. Leanne loves her job, her cats—and herself. So I'm not surprised that she's injected this same joie de vivre into her beauty sessions with me.

Our first project was Leanne's chin, neck, and jowls, which had thickened as she'd entered her forties. We tackled them with liposuction over winter break as Leanne didn't want to pique the curiosity of the children she drives to school—"my kids," as she affectionately calls them. Since then, we've followed a careful plan that suits Leanne's work schedule and her budget. During school time, we stick to no-recovery procedures, such as Botox for her forehead wrinkles and alternating sessions of salt macrodermabrasion and green tea facials to minimize Leanne's open pores and give her a healthy glow. And during school breaks, I've enhanced her lips with fat injections, lasered away the spider veins on her cheeks and nose, and given her a couple of medium-depth chemical peels to tighten her skin, especially around her eyes and jawline.

The results have been subtle and at the same time spectacular. Nobody Leanne knows has figured out that she's had cosmetic surgery, but she stopped by the other day to excitedly report that a colleague had remarked that she looks younger and more beautiful every time he meets her. Later the same day, one of Leanne's smallest—and therefore most honest—passengers had echoed this sentiment when he'd told her, "You look really pretty!"

When Leanne and I looked at her before and after pictures, I was struck by what had changed. Now her jawline is firm and her neck is swanlike. Her facial redness has been tamed and her open pores are a thing of the past. Leanne has responded to this metamorphosis by growing her hair out into glamorous chestnut waves and sweeping it off her newly Botoxed, wrinkle-free forehead.

But I was also struck by what had not changed. The warmth in her eyes and smile were there before we started, and they're still there now. And that's what makes her truly beautiful. For Leanne and other patients like her, I feel I am simply putting the icing on the cake. I'm taking the beauty that is already inside and simply adding to it to make it a little fuller and more apparent.

It can be difficult to recognize your inner beauty, especially when society is sending you mixed messages and holding you to a standard you can't achieve. I still remember being teased as a schoolgirl in England for my black hair and for my lips, which were too full to conform to the Farrah Fawcett style that was then in fashion. Many of my patients speak of similar experiences. These experiences not only can hinder women from feeling beautiful in later life but also can prevent them from feeling they even deserve to be beautiful.

Robyn, for instance, never felt beautiful as an adult because, she said, "I come from a family of gorgeous women and I was always the ugly duckling."

She was in her mid-fifties and a highly respected operating room nurse at a local hospital. I planned to have my anesthesiologist give her "twilight sleep," a form of light sedation, so she'd be totally comfortable while I treated her face with laser resurfacing to tighten her jowls and remove wrinkles and age spots.

Robyn wanted the procedure, but a part of her felt that she didn't have the right to it, that she wasn't entitled to beauty because she'd always been cast in a different role. Her feelings of unworthiness expressed themselves in the form of fear and shame. "I know this is crazy, but my worst nightmare is that things will go wrong and I'll end up being wheeled into the emergency room in front of everyone I know," she confessed.

Despite this, Robyn was quite determined to go ahead with her laser resurfacing. When she awoke from her "twilight sleep," the first thing she did was flash me a big grin. "No emergency room?" she asked with a laugh.

"No emergency room," I replied, suppressing a smile.

Almost a year later, Robyn tells me that the laser treatment was the best thing she ever did. "It seems like I was waiting for it all my life," she now gushes. We laugh together when we reminisce about her preprocedure butterflies. With her quick wit and sharp intellect, Robyn had always been beautiful inside, but cosmetic surgery allowed her to throw off the "ugly duckling" mantle and become a swan.

Feeling good about yourself begins with locating your inner beauty. Ageless, infinite, and divine, this beauty exists within all of us. I believe the best way to tap into it is through meditation.

My personal experience with meditation has been very positive. I consider any activities that allow me to distance myself temporarily from the outside world and to elevate my mind to a higher plane to be meditative. This encompasses not only conventional meditation but also Indian classical singing and even a good workout. All these activities give me a sense of well-being and inner peace. Research shows that I'm not alone. Those who participate in either conventional meditation or aerobic exercise feel more able to cope with life in general and feel very positive about the value of these meditative activities in their lives.

I consider it the greatest compliment when my patients comment that I project an aura of tranquillity. And I will never forget returning a telephone call a couple of years ago to a prospective patient, who told me, "You have the most soothing voice I've ever heard. I'm going to make an appointment with you just so I can meet the owner of that voice!"

I think it's worthwhile for everyone to give conventional meditation a try. This chapter contains the first four of seven meditations that show you how to locate, develop and project your inner beauty. With practice, you'll be able to visualize the clarity and compassion of your inner beauty effortlessly. (See The Gift of Meditation on page 86 and Meditations 1 and 2 on pages 88 and 90.)

Principle 2: Get Past the Ordeal by Mirror

Once you've used Meditations 3 and 4 (see pages 92 and 96) to make friends with your mirror, I want you to go all the way and banish from your life the Ordeal by Mirror, the compulsion that drives you to root out your tiny imperfections and then to feel guilt and shame when you see your reflection as inadequate.

Walk into the ladies' powder room of any good restaurant and you'll see the Ordeal by Mirror at work. We see women bemoaning their faults so commonly that we probably don't even notice it anymore. It's rare to hear them express contentment with how they look. Here's a recent sampling from my restroom visits.

"My hair's such a mess today."

"I can't believe I had to break out just before this date."

"I need Botox—real bad."

At best, the atmosphere in the ladies' room is businesslike. At worst, the tension is almost palpable. The expressions on our faces as we preen tell the same story. There's the woman in the corner, subduing her hair with fierce brush strokes; her grim-faced companion, touching up her lipstick; and, next to her, a younger woman who sighs as she reapplies concealer to her blemishes. The message is clear: being beautiful is hard work, and it's no fun.

I want you to have fun being beautiful. I want you to be able to look in the mirror without feeling a rush of disappointment or inadequacy. And, ultimately, I want you to look beyond the two dimensions of your face that the mirror reflects and see your face as something more profound: the reflection of your inner soul. The first step in doing this is to get rid of the negative feelings that cloud your vision of yourself.

I believe that the only practical way to get beyond a force as powerful and insidious as the Ordeal by Mirror is to work from both the inside and the outside. Generally, we have no difficulty in appreciating the value of working from the inside, of looking within ourselves to discover a deeper truth. But what we do sometimes find hard to recognize is that

(continued on page 94)

The Gift of Meditation

Our nonstop world can prove a challenging environment for delving into matters of the spirit. You're expected to assimilate so much data just by being awake in the 21st century that your conscious mind is usually occupied by your ever-changing thoughts. The aim of meditation is to purposefully transcend this stream of distracting thoughts and to focus on what is constant and unchanging within you.

I can often sense whether someone meditates regularly; her serenity radiates out, smoothing lines and furrows. It's fascinating to watch others meditate and to see the transformation in their faces. Meditation is truly the journey of a lifetime, as you turn your mind inward and dive deep within you to discover the most exciting destination of all, your inner Self. I've capitalized "Self" throughout this book because I want to evoke the concept of your transcendent soul, the source of your ageless beauty, rather than narcissistic or selfish concepts. Successful meditation breaks the barrier between your external persona and your inner Self. I cannot recommend it highly enough.

How do you know that your inner Self exists? Close your eyes and strive to remove outside distractions. What you sense is a feeling of consciousness or being. You sense different parts of your body and are aware of your thoughts and the mind that produces them. Perhaps you also perceive your body and mind to be distinct from an element deep within you, that aspect that gives you your sense of yourself and makes you *you*. This element is your inner Self, which is inseparable from your personal identity. Unlike your body and mind, your inner Self is eternally unchanging. Your body and mind are concrete elements, while your inner Self is abstract.

Learning to focus on an abstract inner Self during meditation is difficult. I've found it much easier to visualize my inner Self in a concrete form. In the meditations, I ask you to visualize your inner Self as a constantly glowing flame. You will visualize the stream of thoughts that distract you as a stream of smoke obscuring the flame.

Fire doesn't speak to everyone. If the image of your inner Self as a flame leaves you cold, try visualizing it as a pool of tranquil water instead. Focus on its depth, stillness and immutability. Or imagine the steady rhythm of a flowing river, removing all distractions as it washes over your senses. There is no one right way to meditate and I hope you'll enjoy experimenting with different images to find what works best for you.

A developed inner Self emits a steady stream of wisdom. This wisdom is the source of an infinite inner beauty that, when reconnected with your external persona, results in enhanced self-esteem, compassion for yourself and for others, confidence, and serenity. In the meditations in this book, the beauty that shines forth from your developed inner Self is represented by the light and warmth of the flame.

These meditations are based upon conventional techniques that require quiet, nondistracting surroundings, a relaxed position with your spine vertical, rhythmic breathing, and a focus point for your mind. I have incorporated some elements of Kundalini yoga, which focuses on visualizing the activation of spiritual energy from the base of your spine. This can be a tremendous source of power in midlife. I have also drawn from methods of body visualization, which are commonly used to activate healing energy in diseased areas

of the body. An ailing self-esteem is the definitive "dis-ease"—as it is a lack of ease with yourself. It can be healed by techniques that inspire self-acceptance and help you to recognize your eternal inner beauty.

I suggest following these general guidelines before beginning the meditations:

- Remove any makeup from your face and arrange your hair so that it does not cover your face.

- Keep a notebook in which you document your experiences during and after each meditation; this can be very helpful in the growing process. You should document your feelings both immediately after the meditation and several hours later.

- Repeat each meditation until you are familiar with it and can consistently achieve the desired results. Then move on to the next meditation. Meditation takes practice, preferably daily. With time, it will become easier and easier to reach the goals of each meditation.

- As you progress through the meditations, continue to practice the previous ones so they stay fresh in your mind.

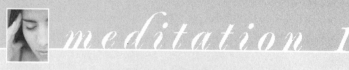

Locating Your Inner Self

This meditation and all that follow begin with your assuming a classical position for meditation, undisturbed by outside distractions and with your spine straight. Rhythmic breathing helps you to relax fully and turn your mind inward. Repetition of words clears your mind and lifts it to a higher spiritual level. Your thoughts are visualized as a stream of smoke. The variation of the smoke's speed and density represents the continuous variation in your thoughts. The casting aside of your distracting thoughts is visualized as stepping through the smoke to discover the flame that represents your inner Self. The light and warmth emanating from the flame represent the inner beauty that emanates from your Self.

As you progress through this meditation, you should feel a wave of relaxation and peace sweep over you. It is common when you begin meditation for random thoughts to enter your mind and distract you. Occasionally, these thoughts may even make you feel uneasy. Do not be discouraged by this. As you gain in experience, intrusive thoughts will become much less frequent and it will become easier to attain the meditative state.

1. Sit comfortably in a quiet place, with your back straight. Your head should be in an unstrained, neutral position. Rest your hands in your lap or clasp them together lightly, and place your legs in a comfortable resting position.

2. Close your eyes gently.

3. Inhale slowly and deeply through your nose while mentally counting to 10.

4. Exhale slowly and fully through your mouth while mentally counting to 10. Feel yourself becoming aware of the thoughts that are passing through your mind.

5. Visualize your thoughts moving across your mind from left to right like a billowing stream of white smoke. Observe how the speed and density of the smoke vary with time.

6. Continue to inhale slowly and deeply through your nose and exhale slowly through your mouth while continuing to focus on the stream of smoke. Repeat to yourself, "I am at peace."

7. Repeat the inhaling and exhaling until you have achieved an effortless breathing rhythm and feel a sense of serenity enveloping you.

8. Feel yourself moving closer and closer to the smoke and finally passing through it.

9. Visualize a constant, glowing orange-red flame behind the smoke screen. This represents your Self: your here-and-now feeling of being or existing.

10. Continue to breathe slowly and deeply until you have achieved an effortless breathing pattern and are no longer aware of the smoke, but only of the flame.

11. Feel the flame's light and warmth radiating toward you.

12. Continue to breathe effortlessly while focusing on the flame and its light and warmth. Feel yourself moving toward the flame and your mind being pulled in toward it.

13. When you feel a sense of serenity enveloping you, focus on it for at least 10 seconds. Then open your eyes slowly.

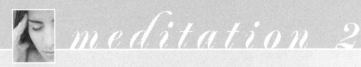
meditation 2

Developing and Projecting
Your Inner Self

This meditation begins with the techniques used in Meditation 1 to cast aside your distracting thoughts and achieve a steady focus on your inner Self. The Self is also known as the spiritual soul. The eyes are the window to the soul and the passage between your Self and your outer persona. You will visualize your inner beauty emanating from your Self and traversing this passage to manifest itself outwardly. You will also visualize the energy of your activated life force rising through you from its source at the base of your spine.

1. Sit comfortably, with your back straight, in a quiet place, at arm's length from a mirror that reflects your entire face and neck. The mirror should be illuminated by natural daylight if possible or with lighting that simulates natural daylight. Your head should be in an unstrained, neutral position. Rest your hands in your lap or clasp them together lightly, and place your legs in a comfortable resting position.

2. Close your eyes gently.

3. Inhale slowly and deeply through your nose while mentally counting to 10.

4. Exhale slowly and fully through your mouth while mentally counting to 10. Feel yourself becoming aware of the thoughts that are passing through your mind.

5. Visualize your thoughts moving across your mind from left to right like a billowing stream of white smoke. Observe how the speed and density of the smoke vary with time; this represents your ever-changing thoughts.

6. Continue to inhale slowly and deeply through your nose again and exhale slowly through your mouth while continuing to focus on the stream of smoke. While doing this, repeat to yourself, "I am at peace."

7. Repeat the inhaling and exhaling until you have achieved an effortless breathing rhythm and feel a sense of serenity enveloping you.

8. Feel yourself moving closer and closer to the smoke and finally passing through it.

9. Visualize a constant, glowing orange-red flame behind the smoke screen. This represents your Self: your here-and-now feeling of being or existing.

10. Continue to breathe slowly and deeply until you have achieved an effortless breathing pattern and are no longer aware of the smoke, but only of the flame.

11. Feel the flame's light and warmth radiating toward you.

12. Continue to breathe effortlessly while focusing on the flame and its light and warmth. Feel yourself moving toward the flame and your mind being pulled in toward it.

13. When you feel a sense of serenity enveloping you, focus on it for at least 10 seconds. Then open your eyes slowly.

14. Look straight ahead at the mirror. Look at each eye for about 2 seconds, then examine your eyes in more detail, noting their shape and the depth and variation of their color. You may find that you tend to focus on one eye in particular; this is determined by which of your eyes is visually dominant. (If you are right-handed, your right eye will usually be the dominant one.)

15. Focus intently on the reflection of your dominant pupil. Look beyond the surface of your pupil and hold your gaze for 10 seconds. During this time, inhale and exhale slowly and deeply, and focus on the mental image of the flame.

16. Close your eyes. Place your fingertips on your temples. Visualize a stream of light and warmth projecting from the flame within you through your pupils. Simultaneously, visualize a stream of light and warmth rising from a flame at the base of your spine and enveloping you. Visualize the light and warmth as representing the clarity and compassion of your inner beauty. Continue to breathe slowly and deeply.

17. Open your eyes slowly.

Seeing Your Face Positively I

The purpose of this meditation is to empower you to see your face in a positive light. Many women are accustomed to focusing on the negative aspects of their appearance. Celebrating your good features—and every face has them—can be an exhilarating and uplifting experience. You may fear that examining your face in minute detail makes you self-indulgent. In fact, you are indulging your Self by taking pleasure in your appearance, but this is not wrong; it is an important step on the path to self-acceptance.

1. Sit comfortably in a quiet place, with your back straight. Your head should be in an unstrained, neutral position. Rest your hands in your lap or clasp them together lightly, and place your legs in a comfortable resting position.

2. Close your eyes gently.

3. Inhale slowly and deeply through your nose while mentally counting to 10.

4. Exhale slowly and fully through your mouth while mentally counting to 10. Feel yourself becoming aware of the thoughts passing through your mind.

5. Visualize your thoughts moving across your mind from left to right like a billowing stream of white smoke. Observe how the speed and density of the smoke vary with time; this represents your ever-changing thoughts.

6. Continue to inhale slowly and deeply through your nose again and exhale slowly through your mouth while continuing to focus on the stream of smoke. While doing this, repeat to yourself, "I am at peace."

7. Repeat the inhaling and exhaling until you have achieved an effortless breathing rhythm and feel a sense of serenity enveloping you.

8. Feel yourself moving closer and closer to the smoke and finally passing through it.

9. Visualize a constant, glowing orange-red flame behind the smoke screen. This represents your Self: your here-and-now feeling of being or existing.

10. Continue to breathe slowly and deeply until you have achieved an effortless breathing pattern and are no longer aware of the smoke, but only of the flame.

11. Feel the flame's light and warmth radiating toward you. This represents your consciousness: the life and energy that emanates from your Self.

12. Continue to breathe effortlessly while focusing on the flame and its light and warmth. Feel yourself moving toward the flame and your mind being pulled in toward it.

13. When you feel a sense of serenity enveloping you, focus on it for at least 10 seconds. Then open your eyes slowly.

14. Open your eyes slowly and look at your whole face and neck in the mirror as if you were seeing them for the first time. Note the expression on your face. As you examine each area in turn, try to imprint its image upon your memory. If you begin to experience negative feelings about your appearance or feel uneasy during the self-appraisal, repeat steps 3 and 4 until the feeling of calmness returns. When performing the self-appraisal, try to do so objectively, as if you were observing a painting or sculpture of another person.

15. Examine the skin surrounding your eyes, noting any wrinkles or discolorations but concentrating on your good points—for example, the curve of your eyelashes or how your eyebrows frame your eyes. Vary your distance from the mirror, beginning at arm's length and moving as close as is visually comfortable. Vary the angle of your eyes to the mirror, beginning straight on and then turning your face to each side.

16. Examine your lips when closed and when slightly parted, noting their shape, color, and fullness. Examine the areas surrounding your mouth, noting any wrinkles or furrows but concentrating on your good points. Vary your distance from and angle to the mirror, as in step 15.

17. Examine the rest of your face, as well as your ears and neck, in the same manner: Begin with your forehead, then move to your cheeks, chin, ears, and neck. Note features or signs of aging, but focus on positive aspects—such as beautiful bone structure, unblemished skin, or a shapely neck.

18. Close your eyes for 10 seconds, continuing to breathe slowly and deeply and to focus on the flame within you and the light and warmth it emanates.

19. Open your eyes slowly.

it can work equally well the other way. A change on the outside *can* allow you to feel more positive about yourself inside by making it fun to look in the mirror again. And that's what many of my patients have discovered.

I vividly recall the first time I met Rochelle, who consulted me because she wanted to reduce the discolorations on her face. A government administrator in her early fifties, she had a face that bore the unmistakable signs of a lifetime's experience and wisdom. And, in her own words, she'd always been "tubby."

"That's just me," she said. "I'm built exactly the same way as my mother and my grandmother. I may never be a stick girl, but that's not going to stop me from getting fit."

Rochelle always came to her salt macrodermabrasion sessions with me straight from the gym and still in her workout clothes. As the weeks passed, her improving skin tone kept pace with her muscle tone. During one of our sessions, I was so impressed by her magnetic aura and gaze that I asked her on impulse if she ever meditated.

"Oh, yes," she replied, and she proceeded to tell me all about her yoga classes and her spiritual reading. The force of Rochelle's presence seemed to remain in the examination room long after she had left it that day. As I continued to see her in the ensuing months, I realized that she already understood what I tell so many of my patients: Even physical perfection cannot create self-esteem. Only igniting your inner beauty can empower you to feel comfortable within your own skin. Rochelle had already been happy with herself when she'd come to see me. Harmonizing her outer appearance with her well-developed inner beauty had simply made her happier.

My third and fourth meditations show you how to see your face positively, as the mirror of the infinite beauty that dwells within you. (See Meditations 3 and 4, pages 92 and 96.)

Principle 3: Take Responsibility for Your Own Happiness

It's one thing to realize that you have a right to be beautiful and happy. Taking responsibility for these rights is another thing altogether.

Modern-day Hindu philosophy advises you to visualize your Self as a thermostat, which maintains its equilibrium even in the face of external change, rather than as a thermometer, which reflects every perturbation in its surroundings. The idea is that you need to empower yourself to maintain your happiness "set point," despite life's challenges, because nobody else can do this for you. I find the image of the thermostat helpful and uplifting.

Alternately, think of your inner Self as a lighthouse standing steady with a constant beam despite the buffeting of the surrounding ocean. How powerful it is to envision your inner Self as a sanctum protected from the vagaries of the outer world!

Many of my patients face immense challenges. And their motivation in seeking cosmetic surgery may be to take charge of one aspect of their lives when other aspects are not controllable. Elizabeth, an attorney in her forties, had to leave her thriving law practice to undergo radiation therapy for a brain tumor. "I feel like I lost 2 years of my life," she told me. "I'm not going to lose any more."

Elizabeth had gone completely bald during the radiation therapy, but she was fearless about baring her naked scalp, with its spiky tufts of regrowing hair, to the world. She came to her appointments dressed stylishly, with a beautiful bandanna to match every outfit. Clearly, this woman was not going to lie down and let cancer walk all over her.

Still, one thing bothered her: the tattoos that had been made on her scalp to mark the areas where she needed radiation. They were tiny black dots, no more than 1/4 inch in diameter. But their significance to Elizabeth was infinitely greater than their size. "I know nobody else will see them once my hair comes back," she explained. "But I'll always know they're there."

To Elizabeth, the tattoos were not a part of her. They belonged to "the beast," as she referred to her tumor, and they would always be a reminder of what she'd been through. "That's why I want them off," she said. "I don't care even if I'm left with big scars from removing them. And I don't care how painful it is. I just want them gone."

Happily, I was able to free Elizabeth of her radiation tattoos with no discomfort (other than the mild, transient stinging of a numbing shot) and a minimum of scarring. I simply numbed the tiny pieces of tattooed skin, removed them with a surgical instrument rather like a miniature cookie cutter, and then placed tiny stitches in the surgical sites. The stitches

(continued on page 99)

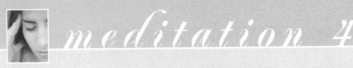
meditation 4

Seeing Your Face Positively II

This meditation expands upon Meditation 3. It introduces touch as a means of enabling you to visualize your face in a positive light. Touch and the application of cream to your face provide sensory stimulation, and you will focus upon the pleasurable sensations this produces. The aim is to awaken positive feelings in you regarding your appearance, by associating the pleasurable sensations experienced during the meditation with your visualization of your face. The visualization of your inner beauty permeating your face paves the way for you to break down the barrier between your outer and inner beauty.

Before you begin, wash your hands and place within reach a jar of noncomedogenic (non-pore-clogging) facial moisturizing cream.

1. Sit comfortably in a quiet place, with your back straight. Your head should be in an unstrained, neutral position. Rest your hands in your lap or clasp them together lightly, and place your legs in a comfortable resting position.

2. Close your eyes gently.

3. Inhale slowly and deeply through your nose while mentally counting to 10.

4. Exhale slowly and fully through your mouth while mentally counting to 10. Feel yourself becoming aware of the thoughts that are passing through your mind.

5. Visualize your thoughts moving across your mind from left to right like a billowing stream of white smoke. Observe how the speed and density of the smoke vary with time; this represents your ever-changing thoughts.

6. Continue to inhale slowly and deeply through your nose and exhale slowly through your mouth while continuing to focus on the stream of smoke. While doing this, repeat to yourself, "I am at peace."

7. Repeat the inhaling and exhaling until you have achieved an effortless breathing rhythm and feel a sense of serenity enveloping you.

8. Feel yourself moving closer and closer to the smoke and finally passing through it.

9. Visualize a constant, glowing orange-red flame behind the smoke screen. This represents your Self: your here-and-now feeling of being or existing.

10. Continue to breathe slowly and deeply until you have achieved an effortless breathing pattern and are no longer aware of the smoke, but only of the flame.

11. Feel the flame's light and warmth radiating toward you. This represents your consciousness: the life and energy that emanates from your Self.

12. Continue to breathe effortlessly while focusing on the flame and its light and warmth. Feel yourself moving toward the flame and your mind being pulled in toward it.

13. When you feel a sense of serenity enveloping you, focus on it for at least 10 seconds. Then open your eyes slowly.

14. Look at your whole face and neck in the mirror as if you were seeing them for the first time. Examine your eyes and the skin around them, your mouth and surrounding areas, and then the rest of your face. Continue to breathe slowly and deeply.

15. Close your eyes. Place your hands lightly on your face so that the fingertips span your forehead. With slow, gentle sweeping motions, touch your face and neck, concentrating on the texture, softness, and warmth of your skin; the curve of your cheekbones, nose, and chin; the curve and fullness of your eyebrows and lips; the fullness and softness of your earlobes; and the length of your neck. Maintain contact between your hands and your skin during this step. As you feel each area, try to

Continued on page 98

recall the visual memory of it, and inhale and exhale deeply as in steps 3 and 4. Try touching your skin in different ways, varying the pressure, speed, and pattern of your touches.

16. Remove your fingertips from your face. Clasp your hands or place them comfortably in your lap. For 10 seconds, continue to breathe slowly and deeply and to focus on the flame within you and the light and warmth it emanates.

17. Open your eyes slowly. Apply facial moisturizing cream to your forehead with your fingertips. Massage the cream over your face and neck, noting the sensations as your hands touch different areas of your skin and maintaining contact between your hands and skin.

18. Close your eyes gently and recall the visual memory of each area as you touch it. Breathe deeply and fully. Finish by holding your fingertips lightly to your temples for 10 seconds, feeling the coolness of your fingertips against your skin.

19. Remove your hands from your skin and rest them comfortably in your lap or clasp them together lightly. Focus on the flame within you and its light and warmth, breathing deeply and fully as in steps 3 and 4. Visualize each area of your face and neck in turn, and feel the light and warmth permeating it. While doing this, repeat to yourself, "I am at peace." When you are breathing effortlessly and you feel enveloped in serenity, open your eyes.

healed beautifully, and even before Elizabeth's hair grew back, they could hardly be seen.

Elizabeth is one of those people who see the silver lining in even the darkest cloud. She loved her new hair—not just because it covered up the previously tattooed areas but also because it was irresistibly thick and wavy.

"I have to stop people from running their fingers through it," she told me proudly. "Forty years of being a straight-haired gal, and now I can throw my heated rollers away!"

(I've seen hair transformation of this type in a few patients besides Elizabeth. When hair appears sporting a new personality, to surprise and delight its owner, it's not only fascinating; it's also awe-inspiring—because there's no medical explanation for it. So many of the wonders of our own biology are still a mystery to us.)

On the face of it, you might find it illogical that a woman stricken with a serious illness would be preoccupied with a seemingly trivial cosmetic issue. But in fact this is a healthy impulse. Elizabeth stayed happy throughout and after her ordeal because she was able to dissociate herself from the terrifying events that threatened to take over and rob her of her life. She chose to focus instead on a smaller issue, a part of her life she could control. By ridding herself of the tattoos, she was symbolically ridding herself of the tumor they represented. I was utterly inspired to see how the removal of a few fragments of skin, no bigger in total than my thumbnail, could transform Elizabeth's quality of life.

Was Elizabeth in denial about her illness? I don't think so. What she did was to analyze her situation, to choose to be happy despite it, and to take positive steps to change what she *could* control.

You don't need to be a cancer survivor to do this. Whether your life challenges are big or small, you can set your internal thermostat and maintain your serenity.

Principle 4: Live in the Present

One often overlooked way to fulfill the beauty within you is to concentrate on living in the present and to avoid basing your actions and feelings on thoughts and memories of the past. Of course, it can be extremely challenging to do this.

Many of my patients are stuck in the past. Some live daily with the memory of themselves as they were. If this memory is glowing, it can be difficult to come to terms with the loss of youthful beauty that inevitably accompanies aging.

Lillian, who was in her late forties, came to see me complaining, "My face is falling." She'd done quite a bit of research on the Internet and arrived armed with a list of questions about various treatment methods. I talked frankly to her about these treatments and also about the other options she had for improving her appearance.

Lillian shook her head emphatically to each of them. Laser resurfacing? "I'm not going to look like a tomato for a week," Lillian told me. Well, then, how about salt macrodermabrasion? "I don't believe that anything with no recovery time could give me any results," she retorted. And so it went on, with Lillian objecting to every rejuvenation option she'd come in search of.

It was Lillian's closing comment that was most revealing: "When I look in the mirror now, I just feel disgusted. I can't even bear to look at pictures of myself when I was younger and had it all."

Lillian's indelible memories of her former beauty were clearly going to prevent her from achieving the beauty she wanted in midlife. She was afraid that whatever she did, she'd only be a pale imitation of what she'd been. Lillian and I talked about this at length, and in the end we decided that it was best that I didn't treat her at all. Despite her protestations to the contrary, I didn't feel she'd be happy with whatever I did, however well I did it.

Sometimes, past memories may be negative—how you were teased for your acne or your prominent nose or your unconventional looks. These negative memories can profoundly disturb your inner peace, and you must let go of them if you want to achieve true inner beauty.

Some remember life not as it was, but as it could have been. Roma was a 30-something whose attractive face was dominated by hundreds of deep pockmarks on her cheeks and forehead. At first glance, you might think these were due to severe adolescent acne. But in fact Roma had lived with them far longer. As a toddler, she reached for a bottle of caustic drain cleaner and it spilled on her face.

Roma first consulted me for an unrelated skin problem. But as she followed up and got to know me better, she began to open up about her face, and we talked about what could be done. I recommended surgical removal of the pockmarks by essentially the same method I'd used to remove Elizabeth's radiation tattoos. I would cut out each pockmark and then put the skin back together with stitches finer than human hairs, a painstaking process that would take several hours. When I was done, Roma would be left with a tiny, thin scar line at each place where a pockmark had been—hardly a perfect result, but infinitely better than the pockmarks. I could then improve, but not remove, these surgical scars with laser treatments.

Roma's response was enthusiastic; she wanted to get started on treatment as soon as possible. But as I discussed the results she could expect, I became more and more concerned. Roma was listening to me, but she didn't seem to hear me. I wanted her to understand that the best she could hope for, even with the advanced technology I would use, was improvement, not perfection. I couldn't predict the exact degree of the improvement because this didn't depend just on me and my work. It would also depend on how Roma's skin healed, which was not completely in my control.

"But you have to understand how excited I am about this," Roma told me, her words coming thick and fast and her eyes gleaming with anticipation. "This is my chance to finally have normal skin."

"It all depends on your definition of 'normal,'" I warned her. "All I can promise you is that your face will look better to some extent."

Who could blame a young woman who'd lived with a disfiguring deformity for as long as she could remember for dreaming of a rosier future? I certainly didn't. But cosmetic surgery can't be built on dreams. It must rest on a solid foundation of reality, or else it all comes tumbling down. I worried that Roma's dreams of a scar-free future would be shattered by the actual surgery, with devastating results to her psyche.

So we compromised. I didn't rush Roma into full-blown surgery. Instead, we started with a test area: a single pockmark, which I cut out, stitched back together, and then lasered over so that she could get a taste of what to expect. Initially, Roma was disappointed, saying that she didn't see much improvement. And I was relieved that we had opted for the test area before taking the full plunge.

A couple of months later she asked me to perform the full scar removal procedure. At that point, she told me, "I'm so glad we did the test first. Now I know what's achievable and what's not. And I know now that if I can't have 100 percent, I can settle for less."

After talking to Roma at length, I realized that this procedure was not mere impulse but a carefully thought out decision. Almost 9 months had passed since Roma and I had first talked. At this point, she'd managed to replace her fantasies of what might have been with the truth of what could be. She could live in, and for, the present without being preoccupied with an unattainable future.

Two years later, Roma's skin is not perfect. When you meet her, you still see the scars from her surgery. But unlike the pockmarks, they are not the *first* thing you see. While her skin will never be her strongest point, it no longer detracts from her sweet smile, her lustrous hair, and her confident gaze. Most important, Roma herself considers the surgery a success.

From the viewpoint of beauty, living in the present means accepting yourself as you are while not denying yourself as you were or might be. My fifth meditation focuses on helping you to see your face positively at different ages. (See Meditation 5, page 130.) Doing so will help you come to terms with how you look now.

Principle 5: Surround Yourself with Beauty

Surrounding yourself with beauty—both tangible and intangible—is a time-honored technique for nurturing your soul. Keep living plants and animals in your home. Clothe yourself with beautiful garments—or, rather, garments that make you feel beautiful. Keep company with people who elevate you rather than bring you down—people who love you and show their love.

Sylvia clearly knew how to do this. She had retired from her administrative job with the federal government a few years previously and was now in her late fifties. Sylvia always enjoyed the small projects she and her husband took on during their spare time, like remodeling their son's bedroom into a den after he left home. After her retirement she was able to pursue this interest and, in fulfilling it, to surround herself with beauty she created herself. She began by taking a few courses in art and in home renovation at her local community center. Soon she was engrossed in her new passion. I was fascinated to see the photographs of her work: the Salvador Dali-esque murals she'd painted on the walls of her living room and bedroom; the textured plaster walls she'd created for her master bathroom. I particularly liked the earthenware urns she'd fashioned, decorated, glazed, and filled with beautiful shrubs to stand, sentrylike, at her front door.

Sylvia had always been slim, of both body and face. As she put it, "I was the only 14-year-old who already had cheekbones!" As she entered her middle years, her chiseled cheeks became more and more gaunt. Sylvia was at a stage in her life where she'd never felt younger or more energetic, and she was distressed that her face did not reflect this but instead made her look tired, pinched, and old.

"My husband says he loves me just the way I am," she said, laughing. "But I want this for myself!"

I was able to fix Sylvia's problems naturally and subtly with fat injections into her cheeks, lips, and smile lines. Then I layered collagen over the fat in her lips to restore their definition and prevent her lipstick from bleeding onto her upper lip. Sylvia and I—and her husband—were enchanted with the results, and she thanked me profusely for "all you've done for me."

"But you've done something for me too," I told her. "I love seeing how you've filled your life with beauty. All I did was add a little more."

Sylvia smiled wryly. "You're right," she replied. "Life is good. But it wasn't always like this."

That's when she told me of her first marriage, at age 17, to a man 10 years older. Sylvia had been a traditional wife, keeping house while her husband went to work, but as the days wore on, she became more and more depressed. In public, her husband was caring and considerate. When they were alone, he constantly made disparaging comments about her appearance, especially her slight physique.

"He'd leave notes for me in the kitchen, telling me to look at myself in the mirror and see how awful I looked," she recalled. "He'd call me from the office and yell at me, screaming, 'For God's sake, eat something today.' After 3 years, I started to feel suicidal and realized I couldn't go on like that."

Sylvia left her husband, and after their divorce, half the people she'd thought were her friends stopped talking to her. She eventually finished the year of high school she'd never completed, and in her early twenties, she enrolled in a local college. When she graduated, a family friend helped her get an entry-level position in the federal government. During those years, she never dated.

"Some of it was guilt over the divorce," she explained, "and some of it was just that I was so much older than the other kids in school. I don't mean just in years but also in life experience."

Sylvia blushed as she remembered how her husband of nearly three decades came into her life. "It was my 28th birthday, and I was going to spend it quietly with my mother. But a couple of the women I worked with insisted that I go out with them to a club. I'd never been in a club in my life! Well, he came up and asked me to dance, and we ended up closing the club down way after midnight. And you know something? In all these years, he's never once criticized how I look—he's always told me I'm beautiful to him however much I weigh."

Sylvia thought it was luck that gave her the happy ending to her story. But I thought differently, and I told her why. Sylvia made her happy ending by her own determination to make something of herself despite her circumstances. As Benjamin Disraeli said, "We make our fortunes and we call them fate."

Whether you believe in fortunes or fate, your life is yours to shape. And the most important and positive decision you can make is to bring beauty into your life.

Principle 6: Do at Least One Thing a Day That Inspires You

We draw oxygen from the air we breathe, but we draw life from our passions. Keep your passions at the center of your days, whatever they may be—music, sports, cooking, reading, or writing. Whatever feeds your soul and makes it sing.

Nora was one of my most contented patients. She talked happily of her inspiring days as a violin teacher, how much it thrilled her each time she brought the gift of music into a child's life and how wonderful it was to share her interests with her husband, a part-time pianist who accompanied Nora's young pupils during their performances.

She grew up in California and spent much of her childhood on the beach. By the time she hit 45, this was all too apparent. Her skin had begun to wrinkle and sag, particularly around her jawline and her eyes and on her neck. The damage you do to your skin in your younger years typically begins to show only as you enter midlife and the mechanisms your body uses to repair the damage slow down.

Nora had been advised by another physician to have a face-lift to tighten the sagging areas, but she told me that she was concerned about the recovery time.

"I can't stop teaching for several weeks. What would the children do? And the doctor told me I can't even play the violin myself for a month because my face will be bruised and sore. That would drive me crazy!"

Equally important, Nora was not happy with the before and after photos the doctor had shown her. "It was so obvious that the patients had had cosmetic surgery," she explained. "They looked completely different; their eyes were a different shape, and they had that overtightened look I really hate! I don't want to change the way I look. I still want to look like me."

Although Nora's skin was loose, it was not hanging in deep folds. In my opinion, she didn't need a face-lift to achieve the results she wanted. And sure enough, I was able to tighten it effectively and also to improve her wrinkles and discolorations with laser resurfacing of her face and neck.

I asked Nora to bring her favorite music with her on the day of her surgery, and I lasered away her sun damage with the sweet strains of a Vivaldi concerto—also my favorite!—playing in the background. Within 8 days, Nora was back to playing and teaching. And she was so delighted with the results that she hugged me during one of her follow-up visits and thanked me for putting the song on her face that she had in her heart.

part three

Linking Inner and Outer Beauty

chapter seven

The Curses of Aging— and What They Do to Your Skin

I'm tired of all this nonsense about beauty being only skin-deep. That's deep enough. What do you want—an adorable pancreas?

—Jean Kerr

If I asked you to name one of your important body organs, you'd probably mention your heart, your liver, or your lungs. It's quite likely that you might not even think of your skin. Considering how much time and money most of us spend on our skin, it's amazing how few of us understand its basic anatomy or function.

Your skin acts as a physical barrier between you and your environment, protecting your body beneath from injury and infection. It shields you from sun damage, holds in moisture, and controls your body temperature. And your skin acts as a psychological barrier too—think of our description of someone who breaches that barrier as "getting under our skin." Depending on how easily our feelings are affected by the outside world, we can be either thick- or thin-skinned.

From the earliest age, your skin is the most obvious hallmark of your individuality and a major indicator of your state of health. At my English medical school, the physical evaluation of a patient was considered to be all-important. This evaluation always began with a skin examination, which alone was often sufficient to make the patient's diagnosis. Every medical illness known has telltale manifestations in your skin or its related organs, your hair, your mouth, and your nails. Take anemia, which is characterized by pale skin and lips; thin, brittle hair; and weak, concave nails. Or the yellow, jaundiced complexion, flushed palms, spider veins, and discolored nails of liver disease. This early emphasis on the skin as the most visual aspect of medicine fueled my fascination with the study of dermatology.

Constantly on display, infinitely vulnerable, your skin is the meeting point between yourself and the outside world. Realistically, it should hardly surprise anyone that skin arouses strong feelings in us. Even so, physicians of other specialties often scratch their heads in puzzlement as they try to understand the powerful emotions unleashed when something goes wrong with a patient's skin.

"It's just a few little scars on her cheeks. I can't imagine why she's so upset; she was crying about it in my office," said an otherwise empathetic internist of the patient he referred to me recently.

"She's totally obsessed," said another, about a woman who'd spent 6 months and most of her savings traveling around the country in an attempt to find out why she was losing her hair.

I find it perfectly normal for your reaction to be out of proportion to the actual physical extent of your skin or hair problem, precisely because what's happening physically is not the only issue. We have such an emotional connection to our skin and hair that it can be very distressing when something goes wrong, whether it's an injury, an acne breakout, or the first signs of aging. If you've yearned since childhood for movie idol skin or hair or other vestiges of glass box beauty, falling short is much more than a mere aesthetic concern—it's a miserable failure that calls your femininity into question.

And it's a failure that cannot be concealed. You can disguise your figure flaws with a well-placed swathe of fabric. But when you fail to achieve "good" skin and hair—or lose them with age—your weakness is exposed to every casual passerby. Unless you've suffered firsthand, it may be difficult for you to understand how traumatic the shame of imperfection can be and how it can paralyze the sufferer into inaction. You often can't see it even in those you're closest to—because they won't let you.

Ashley was a 21-year-old prelaw student who'd had severe acne since age 13. She came to see me at the urging of her mother, who told me that Ashley had always acted as if the acne didn't bother her. But the years of frustration and shame came tumbling out of her when we were alone in the exam room. She interrupted my discussion of treatment options to ask me why I didn't "just save us all the trouble and cut my head off."

An essential part of your beauty strategy at any age is to learn to be at peace with your skin, despite its flaws and the changes it undergoes with time.

A Guided Tour of Your Skin

Before we discuss the curses of aging and what they can do to your skin, I'm going to take you on a brief guided tour of your body's largest and most fascinating organ. To use a savory image, you might think of your skin as being rather like lasagna, with each layer's having a unique structure and purpose.

The Epidermis

The outermost layer of your skin is called the epidermis. It is itself composed of four layers. The innermost, the basal layer, continuously generates living cells that move up progressively through the other three layers of the epidermis. As the cells move up, they become flattened, connect to one another, and produce and accumulate a protein called keratin.

By the time the cells reach the outermost layer, which is known as the stratum corneum, they form a compacted mass of dead cells filled with keratin. A cell takes about 14 days to make the journey from the basal layer to the stratum corneum. The cell then takes another 14 days or so to move up through the stratum corneum to the surface of your skin, where it is sloughed off. The stratum corneum forms a protective barrier for your skin, which shields it from infections, irritating chemicals, and the sun, and prevents moisture loss.

The rate at which the epidermis generates living cells is controlled precisely to match the rate at which dead cells are shed from the skin surface. This precise control makes your epidermis amazingly adaptable to the many challenges it faces as your body's frontline defense. For instance, if your skin is injured, your epidermis produces new, living cells at a faster rate so that the injury heals.

If you look at your epidermis under a microscope, you'll also see some other cells. There are pigment cells, known as melanocytes, in the basal layer. These produce melanin, the protein that gives your skin its color. A little nearer the surface of your skin, you'll see Langerhans cells, which defend your skin (and hence your whole body) from infection by activating your body's immune system when it's needed.

The important point to grasp from the complicated processes going on in the epidermis is that your skin is a naturally self-exfoliating organ. That is, cells are continuously being shed from your skin's surface and being replaced by fresh, new cells.

Visit the cosmetics counters of any department store, and you'll be assailed with innumerable products that promise to "exfoliate" your skin. Talk to any of the white-coated ladies behind these counters, and they'll assure you that an exfoliating product is a vital component of your skin care regimen. But, the simple truth is, many of the exfoliating scrubs you're exhorted to buy can do more harm than good.

When Xiaoshi came to see me, she was in tears. Her wedding was a mere 3 weeks away, and her face was a mess. It had all started when she'd visited a well-known cosmetics counter at an upscale department store 4 weeks previously, looking for a regimen to get her blemish-prone skin into good shape for her wedding. She was told that her skin was "combination to oily" and went home with a cleanser, toner, weekly exfoliating facial scrub, and six other products.

Within a week, Xiaoshi noticed flaking skin on her cheeks and nose. When she returned to the cosmetics counter, she was told that this was because she had too much surface dead skin and that she needed more exfoliation to remove it. She was told to use the facial scrub every day, instead of once a week.

"I've been following the advice faithfully, but the dead skin is still there," Xiaoshi wailed.

By now, Xiaoshi's nose and cheeks were covered with white scales and stung even when she washed them with plain water. As I looked beneath the scaling and saw redness, the diagnosis became clear. Xiaoshi had eczema, a condition caused by the products she'd been using. The more she'd scrubbed her skin, the drier and scalier it had become—and the more she'd scrubbed in a vain attempt to remove the scales. The problem could be solved only by breaking this vicious cycle of skin scrubbing and irritation.

The first step was for Xiaoshi to stop using all of her products. I prescribed a nondrying, soap-free cleanser and a non-pore-clogging moisturizer to rehydrate her skin, and a cortisone-like cream to relieve the eczema. Within 10 days, the redness and scaling were gone, and Xiaoshi was smiling again in anticipation of her wedding photos.

The Dermis

The dermis is the layer lying beneath your epidermis. It contains the essential proteins collagen and elastin, which form collagen and elastic fibers, the structural scaffold of your skin. These collagen and elastic fibers keep your skin firm and resilient. See their effects for yourself: Pinch up the skin on the back of your hand and let it go, and watch your skin snap back into place.

The collagen and elastic fibers in your dermis are embedded in a water-retaining gel known as ground substance. New collagen is constantly produced and old collagen is constantly broken down in your dermis.

Between the collagen and elastic fibers lie hair follicles, from which your hairs originate, and oil-producing glands, which release sebum, your body's natural oil, into the hair follicles. Other glands in your dermis produce sweat, which maintains a steady body temperature. There are nerve endings which detect sensations, including touch, pain, heat, and cold. Your dermis also contains a rich network of blood and related lymphatic vessels that transport nutrients to your skin and remove waste products.

The blood vessels are particularly populous in the upper part of your dermis, which ripples in unison with the lower part of your epidermis.

The junction between your epidermis and dermis is a masterpiece of biological engineering. The ripples greatly increase the area of contact between these two layers of your skin; and the greater the area of contact, the more efficiently the blood vessels in your dermis can provide nutrition to, and remove wastes from, your epidermis.

Think of your dermis as being the support system of your skin. It provides structure, nutrition, temperature control, and waste removal services, and protects your skin by allowing it to detect pain and other harmful stimuli. If your support system is overwhelmed, this can profoundly impair the function of your skin.

Veronica, a corporate public relations consultant in her mid-forties, visited me shortly after a disastrous experience at a well-known local beauty spa. A coworker had given her a holiday gift certificate for a facial there. Veronica, who was more accustomed to putting in 18-hour days in her office than indulging herself, had leaped at the opportunity for a little pampering.

"Everything was fine until the end, when the beautician said she was going to refine my skin with a glycolic acid mask," Veronica recalled. "But my skin started burning intensely about a minute or so after she put that mask on."

Veronica alerted the beautician to her discomfort, but she was told that it was "normal" to feel some tingling or stinging due to the mask. However, when the burning reached almost unbearable heights, Veronica insisted that the mask should be removed. The beautician told her that her skin was "unusually sensitive" and that it might be a little pink for a day or two.

When Veronica got home and checked her face in the mirror, she was alarmed to find that it was not merely pink, but red and raw-looking in some areas. By the time she saw me a couple of days later, these areas had darkened, and her beautiful mocha skin was marred by patchy brownish black discolorations.

Glycolic acid is a great skin rejuvenator, in the right hands and on the right skin. But in Veronica's case, the hands were "wrong"—they belonged to an inexperienced and unsupervised beautician. And her skin was "wrong" too. Glycolic acid should be used with particular caution on any pigmented skin—whether Latin, Asian or, like Veronica's, African-American—because there's a small but definite risk that it will overreact, causing skin discolorations that are tenacious and difficult to fade.

The phenomenon by which irritation of pigmented skin leads to discolorations is all too familiar to many women of color. Even a seemingly trivial skin injury, like a small burn from a curling iron, can metamorphose within a few days into an unsightly brown or black patch. To understand why this occurs, you have to understand the dermis.

When the rippled junction between the epidermis and the dermis is injured, the damaged pigment cells there cannot function normally. As a result, the pigment that would normally be contained within these cells is spilled into the upper part of the dermis. The ever-resourceful dermis calls on specialized cells to mop up this spill. These macrophages literally eat up the spilled pigment and other debris. But they can work only so fast. Skin of color can spill massive amounts of pigment, and it can take months or even longer for the overwhelmed macrophages to clear. In the meantime, the loose pigment discolors the skin. This effect is often compounded by a zone of increased pigmentation in the lower part of the epidermis, which lies next to the dermis.

Veronica's reaction to the glycolic acid mask and the resultant postinflammatory hyperpigmentation couldn't have come at a worse time. She was slated to be a keynote speaker at her company's annual conference a month later. I treated her aggressively with Glyquin, a highly effective prescription hydroquinone fading cream, and Veronica was assiduous about using high-protection sunscreen. By the day of the conference, her skin was much improved. Veronica was able to cover the remaining discolorations with concealer so they did not distract the audience from her eloquent presentation. But it took several more months before she finally regained her previously pristine complexion.

The Subcutaneous Layer

My patients and staff smile when they hear me say that fat is beautiful. But it truly is, in the right places. The third layer of your skin is largely composed of fat, interspersed with blood vessels, nerves, and deep hair follicles, and it has several important functions. The subcutaneous layer insulates your skin from the cold, cushions it from injury, and acts as a source of energy.

Most important from the beauty angle, it provides a supportive "bed" over which your skin is draped. The individual shape of your face is determined by the interplay of your subcutaneous layer with the bones that lie beneath. Run your fingers over your face and you'll understand how this interplay varies in different areas of your face. The shape of your forehead and nose are largely determined by the bones that form them, while the contours of your cheeks and your lips depend on the arrangement of the underlying fat.

To some extent, this arrangement is hereditary. Some of us are born to chubbier cheeks or fuller lips. And to some extent, it depends on your total body fat; if you gain a few pounds, some of it will find its way onto your face. Your subcutaneous layer is not so affected by the external environment as your epidermis and dermis, simply because it's distanced from it. But there are times when what we do on the outside assaults the deepest layer of our skin directly.

Amelia, a postgraduate student in her late twenties, had always been quite disciplined about not picking at her skin. So even she didn't fully understand what made her break her lifelong rule so drastically.

"There was something about this particular zit," she mused, shaking her head in disbelief. "I don't know why it bothered me so much, except it was so red and big and stuck right there on top of my nose. I felt like a rhino; I could see this horn between my eyes every time I looked down. And I had a big date that weekend."

Amelia squeezed her acne cyst with a vengeance, and she even poked a sewing needle into it in an attempt to deflate it. She managed to free herself of the annoying pimple, but ended up with a jagged hole in its place. She canceled her date and came into my office the following Monday, her eyes red from lack of sleep.

"Just tell me I won't be scarred for life," she pleaded as I examined her.

I sighed as I replied, "Amelia, you're going to have a scar when this heals; the injury goes all the way down to the fat layer, which is pretty thin on your forehead. First, we have to get this thing healed, which is going to take several weeks because it's so deep. Then I have to see what the scar looks like to figure out how to make it as invisible as possible."

Amelia suppressed a sob. "But how horrible will the scar be?" she gasped. "Is it going to be really big?"

I sighed again. I wished I could settle Amelia's mind by reassuring her that the scar would not be that bad or by telling her which methods I would use to improve it. But either of these options required a certainty I just didn't have at that point. How well the scar healed—or even exactly how it healed—depended to a large extent on the repair mechanisms of Amelia's skin.

I could and did give her skin the best environment for healing: prescription Bactroban antibiotic ointment, covered at all times by a dressing. Contrary to popular belief, wounds heal better when they're kept moist, not when they're dried out. But the rest was a matter of time and crossed fingers.

Amelia called my office in a panic several times in the ensuing weeks. From her point of view, the wait was interminable and the uncertainty was torture. But finally she began to see results, and ultimately, the scar was as good as I could have hoped for. It was ½ inch or so long and ¼ inch wide, slightly caved in but not markedly so. The scar extended through the dermis to the subcutaneous fat layer.

Six weeks after I cut it out and stitched the surrounding skin back together, all Amelia had to show for her trauma was a hair-thin scar line between her eyebrows. With time, Retin-A, and a little surface sanding, that all but disappeared. Such are the everyday miracles of your skin.

How Your Skin Ages

The changes you see in your skin as you age are the visible signs of its declining function. These changes begin in your thirties and become more pronounced with each passing decade. Dermatology textbooks frequently describe skin's aging as a gradual, progressive process. We can definitely see under the microscope how many of your skin's functions deteriorate in a continuous manner.

Nevertheless, I think we're all familiar with the sensation that many of the aging changes that we witness with our own eyes occur in fits and starts, not incrementally. Time and time again, a woman will point out a sunspot or a wrinkle or a spider vein and tell me authoritatively, "This wasn't here 6 months ago." And I believe her because I've seen it happen repeatedly, particularly to women around the time of menopause.

In all honesty, there's a lot about the aging process that we still don't understand, and at this stage of our knowledge, we may be guilty of over-simplifying the story. A sunspot may start as an imperceptible discoloration, and you may notice it only on the day that it reaches a particular degree of darkness, even if it was there for months or years before. But does this apply to all aspects of aging? Or are there some aspects that occur suddenly, when that last straw (or cell) breaks the camel's back? If this type of aging truly exists, we could compare it to a rope's being continuously pulled, appearing quite robust until the moment when it snaps without warning.

It's vitally important that your doctor listen to you and try not to impose her concepts of how your skin "should" be aging upon your observations of what's actually happening. Scientific theory is fine, provided it helps to illuminate the problems rather than blind us to solutions.

As we go along here, I'm going to be brutally blunt about what happens to your skin and hair with time. I want to give you our current understanding of how and why it happens, but I don't want you to slip into despair as *you* recognize some of the changes you're seeing and feeling in your own face. The whole purpose of describing these changes is so that we can later discuss what you can do about them.

Roughness and Dryness

These common problems are due primarily to changes in the epidermis and dermis. Your epidermis becomes less efficient at the process of renewing itself by producing new cells and shedding the old, dead ones to reveal the newer, smoother cells beneath. This is partly due to a flattening of the junction between your epidermis and your dermis, which reduces the amount of nutrition that can reach your epidermis from the blood vessels in your dermis. The accumulated dead cells on your skin surface make it look and feel rough. An extreme accumulation of dead cells causes yellow, tan, or brown warty growths that seem to stick on top of your skin. These seborrheic keratoses are quite benign, but not particularly appealing.

Your aging epidermis also becomes less watertight, and the oil glands in your dermis produce progressively less sebum, your skin's natural oil. These changes make your skin less efficient at preventing water loss and more likely to dry out. Typically, dryness develops around the eyes, on the cheeks, and on the neck—where it has the unfortunate effect of making wrinkles more noticeable.

Gauntness

As we enter our thirties and beyond, we all tend to lose fat from our faces—even if we're gaining it elsewhere. The wry French observation that every woman must choose at some point between her face and her derrière is rooted in a cruel fact of life. Maintain a body weight that conforms to today's attenuated ideals of beauty, and your face is likely to become more and more gaunt as the years pass. To see the faces that accompany a more realistic female physique, look at Botticelli's Venus, or the rounded cheeks of the women in ancient Indian temple sculptures, or the contestants in the modern-day Ms. Black International Pageant.

As your facial fat diminishes, your cheekbones become less prominent and appear to drop. Your cheeks and the zone below your eyes may acquire a hollowed-out appearance. Your nose often becomes more prominent and may start to look beaky, as what little fat there was on it disappears. And your smile lines, which run from the sides of your face to the corners of your mouth, deepen. These changes are paralleled on the backs of your hands, which start to look bony and veined as they lose fat.

Discolorations

Your overall skin tone becomes lighter as you age, due to a steady decrease in the number of pigment cells in your epidermis. You may also develop small areas of dramatic pigment loss, especially in sun-exposed areas like your hands, arms, and legs; these appear as white confetti-like spots.

However, what you'll probably notice more are dark spots, the result of uncontrolled proliferation of pigment cells. These age spots or sunspots (also known rather misleadingly as liver spots) spring up on your face and other sun-exposed areas. It's not just age but also cumulative sun damage over many years that makes these pigment cells behave abnormally. You may also see larger patches of discoloration, especially on your face. These may be brought on or worsened by female hormones if you are pregnant, take the Pill, or are on hormone therapy.

We've all seen the extreme end of this spectrum: the habitual sun worshipers whose faces, arms, and chests are covered with irregular brown blotches. When my daughter was 3 years old, she watched a line of passengers waiting to board a plane to Florida, and asked me why there were so many "leopard ladies" at the airport. Out of the mouths of babes . . .

Looseness

Age weakens the collagen fibers in your dermis by interfering with the finely tuned cycle of collagen formation and breakdown. Your elastic fibers decrease in number and become thinner. As these changes cause your skin to lose strength and flexibility, it becomes more vulnerable to the forces of gravity and begins to sag and form wrinkles. For Grace, as with many other women in their fifties, this was most noticeable at her jawline, around her eyes and mouth, and on her neck. As a result, she'd developed jowls, sagging eyelids, bags under her eyes, deepened smile lines, and a crepey neck.

Dilated Veins

Your weakened collagen and elastic fibers are a poor support for the blood vessels in your dermis. These blood vessels are under constant pressure from the blood within them. Without a counterbalancing pressure from the dermis surrounding them, they tend to dilate and form thread-like red or purple spider veins or red spots. Nicole spent every summer at the beach in her twenties and started to notice spider veins from her mid-thirties onward, especially on her nose and cheeks, where sun exposure had contributed to the weakening of her collagen and elastic tissue.

Thinning Hair

Hair is a lose–lose proposition as you get older. You lose it where you want it—in your scalp. And you gain it where you don't—on your face. Witness the chin hairs that are the bane of many a midlife woman's existence. This combination of unpleasantness occurs because your hair follicles are sensitive to your altered levels of female and male hormones before, during, and after menopause.

You may be losing hair for other reasons too. Midlife stress and heredity also contribute to hair shedding. Ingrid, who first noticed her hair was thinning around the time she turned 40, had several female and male relations on her mother's side of the family who had the same problem. The good news is that even if you've inherited the predisposition to hair loss, it's highly unlikely that you'll go bald, as men do. In women, the hair loss tends to be more diffuse, so that you have some degree of thinning over your whole scalp—much easier to hide than a glowing dome.

Gray hair can strike at any point from your twenties onward. I've even seen a few women who began to gray in their teens. This change is largely hereditary and happens because your hair loses pigment cells with age, just as your skin does.

Acne and Rosacea

Acne is not the preserve of hormone-plagued teenagers; at least half of my acne patients are women age 30 and older. During midlife's hormonal shifts, acne around your mouth, chin, and jawline and even on your neck is quite common. Deep red nodules or cysts are not only unsightly; they can be painful.

Rosacea is an adult form of acne that has three features: acne pimples, redness and easy flushing of your nose and cheeks, and spider veins. You may have all three features, only one, or any combination of two. Rosacea has a hereditary basis and seems to be triggered by hormonal shifts. It can be worsened by physical exertion, stress, heat, or cold or by drinking alcohol or caffeine.

I think of acne and rosacea as the Chinese water torture of midlife. Many doctors are surprised that something as "mild" and "normal" as a few premenstrual pimples or a little facial flushing can be so frustrating. But as my patient Karen put it: "What my other doctors don't understand is that the acne's always there. I get a cyst a week or two before my period, and it takes until midcycle for it to go away. By then another cyst is appearing. And the red marks stay for weeks after the cysts have gone. I haven't had one day of clear skin in the past 6 years. Sometimes I just look in the mirror and feel like crying."

You're Not Alone

It's not easy to talk about the changes of aging, even to your best friend. You compare notes about so many aspects of your life—the movie you just saw, the newest restaurant in town, what's happening at home and work. But it takes an enormous show of vulnerability to sit down and discuss your wrinkles. And that's why so many women feel isolated, like it's happening only to them. Rest assured, this is not true. Aging happens to us all.

While this process may happen to different degrees and at different rates for each woman, you are not powerless. You *can* control how you age—and I'm going to show you how.

chapter eight

Walk in Beauty— Lifestyle Choices That Restore Your Beauty

With beauty may I walk
With beauty before me may I walk
With beauty behind me may I walk
With beauty above me may I walk
With beauty all around me may I walk

—Navajo prayer

When I was about 10, I discovered a fascinating book on the shelf in our family room. Titled *101 Ways to Bring Out Your Beauty*, it was incongruously sandwiched between a couple of other paperbacks: *101 Tricks to Make the Most of Your Garden* and *101 Household Hints*. Perhaps the fact that I skipped the home and garden and went straight for beauty was a harbinger of things to come.

101 Ways neatly summarized our understanding of beauty in the 1970s. The chapter in that book that still rings loud and clear in my mind is the one on aging and what changes to expect at each stage of your life. Turning 30 was described as the point at which your first wrinkles began to appear—your first "real" wrinkles, as the book put it, "not the fine lines around your eyes that appear after sunbathing in your twenties and can be banished by a few early nights."

Even today, we're awash with beauty books that enumerate and describe in detail the ways in which your face "will" age in your thirties, forties, and fifties. This defeatist philosophy does nothing to enhance your understanding of the aging process. All it does is to emphasize your powerlessness by encouraging you to simply sit back and watch your face degenerate before your eyes in a preordained manner.

Instead, I want you to have both a broader approach to aging and higher expectations of your ability to slow the process. *101 Ways* and its latter-day descendants attempt to pigeonhole us into stereotypical schedules of aging, when the truth is that no two women age in the same way or at the same rate. There is no fixed age at which your first wrinkles appear, and there's no consistent order or pattern. You can control all these variables to some extent if you live well.

Martha is 73, a lithe and vivacious ex-dancer who professes to eat "a lot of green stuff and not a lot of the red" and still works out at the barre several times a week. Of course she has wrinkles, but far fewer than some women who are 10 or more years younger. Looking at her, with her translucent skin, sparkling hazel eyes, and megawatt smile, you see that she truly walks in beauty.

And so can you. All you need is the knowledge of how your lifestyle can promote or suppress your beauty. There is potential in every aspect of your lifestyle for controlling your rate of aging. Every day, I want you to seize the opportunity to enhance your beauty in the most noninvasive manner, simply by changing the way you live. Don't worry—you don't have to live like a saint to have beautiful skin. If you live consciously in a way that feeds your soul, rather than reflexively feeding your appetites, beauty will follow.

What's Intrinsic and What's Extrinsic?

Open any dermatology textbook or any book on skin written for the general public, and you'll encounter a very basic tenet of aging: the dichotomy of intrinsic aging versus extrinsic aging, two distinctly separate types of aging. Intrinsic aging, or "aging from within," is said to be due to preprogrammed hereditary changes in your skin. Extrinsic aging, or "aging from outside," is said to be due to external factors that can be mitigated. Every book that addresses the issue of aging delves deeply into this dichotomy, dividing your wrinkles into the inevitable and the preventable.

To some extent, this dichotomy does hold true. Each of us has her own aging clock, which determines how fast we start to look older. For proof, take a look around the room at your next high school reunion and see the vast variation in faces. Or read James Clavell's *Shogun*, a novel set in medieval Japan and England. Blackthorne, the hero, is stunned by the contrast between the aging, gray-haired 29-year-old wife he left behind in England and the still youthful Japanese woman of about the same age whom he loves. And he's moved to tears at the thought of what has happened to his wife.

The aging clock is not totally just; only some of our aging differences can be attributed to how we've lived. Some aging is simply inherited, and this is what is called intrinsic aging. We've all seen youthful 40-year-olds, with correspondingly youthful 70-year-old mothers. I've even seen a few—and, I must emphasize, only a few—habitual sun worshipers or smokers who've retained the tautness and smoothness of youthful skin into middle age despite all the odds. Phenomenal inherited skin repair mechanisms must be at work here, because what really determines your rate of aging is how efficiently your skin repairs the damage it sustains on an everyday basis.

Conversely, there's no doubt that controllable extrinsic factors, like sun exposure and smoking, do profoundly affect your rate of aging. Most of what you may think of as "normal" aging is in fact due to the sun.

Nevertheless, I feel that our unquestioning adherence to the dichotomy of extrinsic and intrinsic prevents us from ever truly understanding or coming to terms with the aging process. I've encouraged you to move away from the concept that a beautiful woman must be "born with it" and to instead adopt the attitude that any woman can achieve beauty if she sets her mind to it. Similarly, I don't want you to think of aging as divided into the controllable (extrinsic aging) and the uncontrollable (intrinsic aging). If you think of any aspect of aging as being uncontrollable, you're again falling into the defeatist mindset that a woman who wants to stay youthful has to be "born with it," at least to some extent. So

I'm going to give you some examples of how the dichotomy breaks down.

For years, when I've presented at seminars, I've shown a slide that's supposed to demonstrate the aging effects of the sun. This slide is as familiar to dermatologists as the Statue of Liberty is to New Yorkers. One half of the slide shows a 70-year-old Indian plains woman, her face weathered and furrowed from a lifetime under the blazing sun. On the other half of the slide is a Buddhist monk of the same age who has spent much of his life cloistered indoors. His face is smooth and unlined. Of course, this slide eloquently depicts the damaging effects of the sun upon your skin. But I've come to believe that the slide shows more than that.

Look past the monk's skin and into his eyes, and you see a look of utter tranquillity. Has spiritual fulfillment contributed to his youthful appearance? And if so, is this an intrinsic or extrinsic aging factor? It's something that works from within and thus may be considered intrinsic. But the pursuit of spirituality is not uncontrollable, as intrinsic factors are supposed to be. The monk has made a conscious decision to meditate—it's something he's chosen to change about his environment. By the controllability criterion, spiritual development is an extrinsic factor.

And the waters get muddier when we consider the monk's diet. As a Buddhist monk, he's likely vegetarian, or nearly so. Your diet is something external that you can control—that is, an extrinsic factor. But in the monk's case, his inner spirituality causes him to eat as he does. So we now have to define diet as an extrinsic factor that can be affected by another factor—spirituality—that is either intrinsic or extrinsic, depending on how you look at it. Continue in this vein and all you'll probably get out of the extrinsic–intrinsic dichotomy is a headache.

Think again of the *Shogun* story. Why exactly does the Japanese woman look younger? Is it her Asian ancestry, which is intrinsic? Or is it the fact that she eats and lives better than her louse-infested counterpart in medieval England? Are these extrinsic factors because she controls them? Or are they intrinsic because the way she lives is due to her spiritual philosophy (which is intrinsic or extrinsic, depending on your viewpoint)? At the end of the day, if all this labeling does not help us really understand why she looks younger, why do we do it?

If the division of aging into intrinsic and extrinsic factors doesn't further our understanding of aging in real people, I question the need for that division at all. Dermatologists, like all physicians, love to classify things: Type III melanoma, type II skin, type I antibodies. These classifications are useful up to a point, but they also serve to hide a deeper truth. We define medicine as science when, in truth, it's as much art as science. Dermatology, like every branch of medicine, is the 5,000-piece jigsaw puzzle for which we have only a random half of the pieces. We can fit some of the pieces together with certainty. But we can only speculate on where some of the other pieces belong or what should lie in some of the gaps. This applies particularly to the arenas of beauty and aging, where so much is as yet unknown.

So, for now, let's forget about intrinsic and extrinsic aging and focus instead on the central message: aging is not a passive process during which you stand by helplessly and watch your face and body fall apart. Aging is a process you *can* control. The easiest and most noninvasive way is to modify your lifestyle to eliminate or reduce those factors that are toxic to your beauty and to replace them with positive lifestyle strategies that retard aging.

Taming Those Free Radical Raiders

Think of your lifestyle—what you eat and drink, how you deal with stress, whether you get enough sleep or too much sun—as the bridge between your inner and outer beauty. Living well nourishes your soul, and your inner beauty literally radiates from your face.

Before you can adopt a skin-healthy lifestyle, it's important to identify which habits are toxic to beauty and to understand why. Many of these habits overload your body with harmful chemicals called free radicals.

In the past few decades, there's been a frenzy of scientific research into free radicals and their effects upon our bodies. The major focus of interest is the free radical theory of aging, which states that free radicals are the villains in the aging process. The specific evidence that free radicals are the primary cause of skin aging is quite compelling.

Free radicals are formed by many reactions in your body, and they damage your cells by a process known as oxidation. Your skin, like the other parts of your body, can fight and destroy free radicals through various so-called antioxidant mechanisms. But when your antioxidants are overwhelmed, the result is free radical overload.

Your skin is a major target for free radical overload, for three reasons. First, it has the largest surface area of all your body organs and thus a greater capacity for accumulating free radicals. Second, it has a high metabolic rate. If you peered at your living skin under an extremely high-powered microscope, you'd see a whirlwind of chemical reactions occurring at breakneck speed, resulting in the constant generation of free radicals. Third, many of your skin's components are exquisitely sensitive to free radical damage, including the collagen, elastic, and ground substance that provide all-important structural support. Free radicals damage your skin's DNA, the inherited blueprint that contains the codes for all the characteristics that make your skin uniquely yours, from its color to its resilience, from to how well it fights infections and tumors to how well it regenerates. All this damage from free radicals activates processes within your skin that age it, break it down, and cause the development of tumors.

Laboratory experiments consistently demonstrate the severe damage that free radicals can inflict on skin collagen, elastic, and ground substance. You can easily visualize the resulting skin sagging and wrinkling that would occur if these all-important structural supports break down. Also, by attacking your DNA, free radicals destroy your skin's ability to produce fresh, new collagen, elastic, and ground substance to replace its damaged support system.

Unfortunately, as you get older, you are more likely to develop free radical overload because your body becomes progressively less able to destroy free radicals. One reason for this may be that your pineal gland, a small, cone-shaped structure within your brain, produces less of the hormone melatonin, one of your body's main antioxidants.

The net effect of free radical damage is something of a vicious cycle: Free radical overload ages you, and this aging in turn decreases your body's ability to destroy free radicals, resulting in further free radical overload and further aging The question is, can you control your tendency to develop free radical overload as you get older? I believe you can, by modifying various aspects of your lifestyle, including smoking, stress level, diet, sun exposure, and exercise. You can take direct action against aging and preserve your beauty by minimizing your body's production of free radicals and maximizing your body's antioxidant defense mechanisms.

Make Your Skin a Smoke-Free Zone

My patient Tracy was surprised when I asked her how much she smoked per day.

"But how did you know?" she demanded. "Nobody usually does; I'm really careful to only smoke outdoors so my hair and clothes don't pick up the smell."

But it wasn't my nose that identified Tracy to me as a smoker; it was my eyes. At the tender age of 32, she was already developing the sallow skin discoloration, gaunt cheeks, and wrinkles around her mouth that characterize "smoker's face."

Good blood circulation is essential for healthy skin and hair. If you were to view the multiple layers of your skin under a microscope, you'd be amazed by the plethora of blood vessels in every layer. These blood vessels transport vital nutrients and chemical messengers to the skin while removing harmful toxins. Studies show that smoking decreases blood flow within your skin, thus slowing the delivery of nutrients and the removal of toxic substances. This is one of the reasons that smoking is so destructive to beauty.

Another reason is that smoking damages your skin's elastic fibers. Recent research supports the premise that these effects on blood vessels and elastic fibers are mostly caused by free radicals.

Besides interfering with these critical functions, smoking also increases your risk of developing skin cancers, slows your skin's healing rate, and worsens your hormonal imbalances during perimenopause and menopause. If you smoke, quitting is one of the most important actions you can take to slow your rate of aging.

Besides the outer damage wreaked by smoking—whether firsthand or secondhand—there's also the inner damage to consider. Any addiction serves as a physical and emotional crutch, something you have to lean on to feel whole. You cannot focus on recognizing your inner Self, or on strengthening it, if your next nicotine fix is your major preoccupation.

If you're contemplating cosmetic surgery, you should be doubly motivated to quit since even light smoking hinders skin healing and can

(continued on page 132)

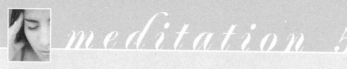

Relaxation and Release from Emotional Crutches

This meditation will help you in your quest to free yourself from any habit that impedes the development of your inner and outer beauty and their reconnection. These habits might include smoking, excessive alcohol or caffeine intake, undesirable dietary habits, or even self-destructive behavior such as picking at your skin or addiction to tanning beds.

You will visualize the power of your inner beauty emanating from your Self and manifesting itself outwardly. You will also visualize the activation and rising of your life force from the base of your spine. You will visualize your inner beauty and life energy protecting you and overpowering the emotional crutch.

I suggest separate meditation sessions for each emotional crutch. You should continue this meditation regularly on a long-term basis.

1. Sit comfortably in a quiet place, with your back straight. Your head should be in an unstrained, neutral position. Rest your hands in your lap or clasp them together lightly and place your legs in a comfortable resting position.

2. Close your eyes gently.

3. Inhale slowly and deeply through your nose while mentally counting to 10.

4. Exhale slowly and fully through your mouth while mentally counting to 10. Feel yourself becoming aware of the thoughts that are passing through your mind.

5. Visualize your thoughts moving across your mind from left to right like a billowing stream of white smoke. Observe how the speed and density of the smoke vary with time; this represents your ever-changing thoughts.

6. Continue to inhale slowly and deeply through your nose again and exhale slowly through your mouth while continuing to focus on the stream of smoke. While doing this, repeat to yourself, "I am at peace."

7. Repeat the inhaling and exhaling until you have achieved an effortless breathing rhythm and feel a sense of serenity enveloping you.

8. Feel yourself moving closer and closer to the smoke and finally passing through it.

9. Visualize a constant, glowing orange-red flame behind the smoke screen. This represents your Self, your here-and-now feeling of being or existing.

10. Continue to breathe slowly and deeply until you have achieved an effortless breathing pattern and are no longer aware of the smoke, but only of the flame.

11. Feel the flame's light and warmth radiating toward you. This represents your consciousness: the life and energy that emanates from your Self.

12. Continue to breathe effortlessly while focusing on the flame and its light and warmth. Feel yourself moving toward the flame and your mind being pulled in toward it. When you feel a sense of serenity enveloping you, focus on it for at least 10 seconds.

13. Keeping your eyes closed and breathing effortlessly, visualize the emotional crutch from which you wish to be released, and picture yourself performing the activity. If you begin to experience negative feelings or feel uneasy during the visualization, repeat the breathing in steps 3 and 4 until the feeling of calmness returns. Try to feel detached from the vision of yourself performing the unwanted activity.

14. Place your fingertips lightly on your temples. Visualize your inner beauty as a stream of light and warmth projecting from the flame within you through the pupils of your eyes and from a flame at the base of your spine. As you do this, continue to breathe slowly and deeply.

15. Visualize the streams of light and warmth enveloping and protecting you. Now visualize the emotional crutch melting away under the force of your inner beauty's light and warmth.

16. Close your eyes for 10 seconds, continuing to breathe slowly and deeply and to focus on the flames and their light and warmth. Feel the power and compassion of your inner beauty continuing to envelop and protect you from the emotional crutch.

17. When you feel a sense of serenity and liberation overwhelming you, open your eyes slowly.

cause poor surgical results. In this chapter, I've included a meditation (see Meditation 5, page 130) to free you from emotional crutches, including smoking. I also urge you to consult your physician to discuss the ever-expanding range of treatments available to help you quit.

Worship Your Skin, Not the Sun

When my patient Laura, who was in her late thirties but looked 10 years older due to her frequent sunbathing bouts, asked me for the three best ways that she could keep aging at bay, my answer was succinct: "Sun protection, sun protection, and sun protection."

If you want to know how the sun has affected *your* skin, look at the inside of your arm, which has had little exposure to the sun. Now look at your face, neck, or chest or the backs of your hands. If they're wrinkled, rough, or discolored, that's sun damage from ultraviolet light exposure, not "normal" aging. So are spider veins and the precancerous red, scaly growths known as actinic keratoses. Are you shocked to learn that the number of wrinkles on your face is directly related to the total hours of sun exposure you've had in your life?

Even if you think you've been "careful" about the sun, the chances are, you've received far more sun exposure than women of previous eras. One reason is changes in lifestyle, which find us spending much more time outdoors, not just on the beach or by the pool but on the tennis court or golf course, in the car, and on the Little League field. The other reason is that the atmospheric ozone layer has thinned dramatically in recent years. Because of this, less of the sun's ultraviolet light is filtered out and more reaches the earth. Scientists have reported holes in the ozone layer since the 1970s. More recently, it's been found that the thinning ozone layer has increased the sunburning ultraviolet light rays reaching Canadians by 7 to 12 percent, depending on the season. We're exposed more and protected less than ever before.

The results are plain to see: an explosion of skin cancers and of premature aging. And the results are equally obvious under the microscope; sun-damaged skin is characterized by degenerated elastic fibers, a drastic loss of collagen and clumped pigment. This shows up as wrinkling, sagging, discolored skin. Scientific evidence points the finger at free radical overload as the cause of sun-induced skin aging.

By her own admission, Phyllis's life was ruled by the sun. In her teens, she'd been one of the baby-oil-and-iodine crowd, seizing every opportunity to darken her always-present tan. As she moved into her thirties, she began to see the effects of her chronic ultraviolet light over-exposure, but this did nothing to dampen her ardor for the sun. By the time she reached 45, she had only a few islands of normal-colored, un-damaged skin left, in areas that she'd never exposed. The rest of her skin was covered with freckles, many of which had merged to form large, ugly discolored patches. The lines around her eyes and mouth made her look years older than she was. Whenever I looked at her, I found it difficult not to remember my daughter's description of "leopard ladies."

When I examined her skin, I pointed out several precancerous growths on her face and body. Phyllis smiled sheepishly.

"I know I shouldn't be doing this, but I can't stop," she declared. "My previous dermatologist used to give me a half-hour lecture every time I saw him and show me really scary pictures of skin cancer. And even my hus-band's fed up. I'm spending hours every weekend lying in the sun or on a tanning bed, and he complains that we never have any time together."

We all love the sun; it gives us a feeling of well-being. Who has not leaped out of bed with a spring in her step as the warm glow of the morning sun illuminated her face? But Phyllis had gone far beyond mere love—she was truly addicted. The sun was destroying her, just as an over-dose of alcohol or drugs would. It was clear that there was no point in my trying to nag her into giving up her habit. Her previous doctor had tried this and failed. In order to help her, I had to first understand her compulsion.

Phyllis had come of age in the era when a tan symbolized health and wealth. And as it turned out, Phyllis had neither as a child. The daughter of a blue-collar family in Maryland, she'd suffered from asthma, which had prevented her from taking part in many physical activities with her peers.

"I was always the one watching from the sidelines," she recalled. "I was never one of the popular girls in junior high. I wasn't a cheerleader and I didn't do sports."

But in high school Phyllis found an entrée into the popular set. She returned from a rare family vacation at the beach with a tan and, she re-called, "Suddenly I looked slim and I looked healthy. Everyone started talking to me."

From then onward, Phyllis dedicated her life to staying bronzed. She'd skip classes in college to lie out in the sun. In her early days as a secretary, she spent much of her pay on tanning beds. When she looked at herself in the mirror, she didn't see the terrible damage the sun was wreaking upon her skin—she saw the unforgettable summer of her 15th year, when Phyllis the also-ran became Phyllis the golden girl. Tanning was what made Phyllis feel beautiful.

We sat down together and looked at the figures. If Phyllis took all the money she'd been spending on tanning, she could use it to visit a salon and have a professional exfoliation and application of sunless tanner once a month.

Phyllis wrinkled up her nose at this. "But I don't care if I look white," she said. "It's not the tanned look I'm after. I just can't stop tanning."

That's when I understood that Phyllis was addicted to the act of tanning, not the effect. If I wanted to help her kick the habit, I needed to find an experience that would provide her with the same relaxation she derived from lying on the tanning bed.

"Then try a facial here in the office," I suggested. "You'll get 1 hour of pampering, and it'll actually help your skin, rather than harming it."

This turned out to be the key. Phyllis loved her facial and soon began coming in regularly for more. She was able to transfer, from the tanning lamp to the steamer, her feelings of being nurtured, loved, and beautiful. And I knew she was free when she let her tanning club membership expire.

A few simple lifestyle modifications can make all the difference in helping forestall the effects of the sun. Avoid hitting the beach, playing outdoor sports, or gardening between 10 and 3. Wear sunscreen every day, all year round. Even on a cloudy day, and even in your car with the windows rolled up, you're getting plenty of exposure to the sun's ultraviolet light. And remember that there's no such thing as a "healthy tan."

Many times, patients will listen to my advice and tell me, "But it's too late; I've spent half my life in the sun." The truth is, it's never too late. Even if you already have significant sun damage, your skin will improve if you cover what you can, avoid excess sun exposure, and use sunscreen.

I consider wearing sunscreen to be an essential part of dressing your skin for aging success. However, I want you to understand some of the controversies surrounding its use. First, be aware that some studies have questioned the value of sunscreen in protecting you from sun-induced aging. The sun protection factor (SPF) number you see emblazoned on your bottle of sunscreen is not as reassuring as it may seem. This number tells you only how well the sunscreen protects you against damage from one type of the sun's ultraviolet rays—UVB—and from the sunburn this causes. A sunscreen with SPF of 15 allows you to stay in the sun without burning for 15 times longer than you could otherwise.

The truth is, sunlight's other type of ultraviolet light—UVA—is far more insidious. Some authorities believe that UVA, capable of causing at least as much skin damage as UVB, is *more* harmful. The problem is, it doesn't burn your skin the way UVB does. So you can be overexposed to UVA and not even know it. Even closed windows in your car or office don't protect you from UVA because it can pass through glass. This has led to concerns that sunscreens could actually *increase* your sun damage and your risk of skin cancers and premature aging. If your sunscreen prevents you from burning, you could be lulled into a false sense of security and actually stay out longer in the sun, during which time you'll soak up more harmful UVA rays. Research shows that children who wear sunscreen tend to spend more time in the sun than children who don't.

So your first strategy is to choose one of the newer sunscreens which not only contains UVB protection, as shown by its SPF, but also is labeled for UVA protection. And take heart from the studies that show that using sunscreen does reduce one's risk of developing precancerous skin growths.

The second issue for you to understand is what the SPF actually means. Women come into my office every day, insisting that they are wearing sunscreen by saying, "My makeup contains it." They're very surprised when I tell them that's not good enough. Or they ask why I recommend a sunscreen with SPF of 25 or above when they've read that anything over an SPF of 15 does not provide additional protection.

You may be surprised to learn just how much sunscreen you have to apply to get the protection that's promised by the SPF label. It's at least 2 ounces, or 4 tablespoons, for your whole body. Scale this down to your face, and that's a teaspoon or two. Try applying this much sunscreen to your face, and you'll probably agree with me and with the studies—virtually nobody uses this much in real life. Most people apply about one-quarter to one-half as much. And if you applied 2 teaspoons of makeup to your face, all you'd be ready for is next Halloween! The average person's application of SPF 15 sunscreen or makeup provides protection equivalent only to SPF 5 or so.

See why using higher-SPF products makes sense? If you apply an inadequate amount of SPF 30 sunscreen to your face, at least you can hope to get SPF 15 out of it. Please think of sun protection in makeup as an addition to the sunscreen you wear beneath it, not a substitute for it. (By the way, correct application of sunscreen also means applying it at least 20 minutes before you go out, so that it has a chance to bind to your skin's surface.)

The third concept for you to grasp is that sunscreen is not the be-all and end-all of sun protection. It's difficult, if not impossible, to apply it evenly to every square inch of your skin; you sweat it off; and it breaks down in the sun. What's more, sunscreen protects you against only ultraviolet light. Some research has even suggested that, in addition to UVA and UVB, regular, visible light—if it's intense enough—is also a risk factor for skin cancer.

The most reliable way to prevent sun damage is to avoid being out in open sunshine when you can and to cover your exposed skin with protective clothing. But be aware that the average summer tee-shirt gives you SPF of only 5 to 9, and less if it's wet. If you're out in the sun a lot, it's worth looking into the lines of clothing that are specially designed to give you SPF values of 30 or above. Use sunscreen in addition to, but not instead of, these measures. And if you hate feeling greased up, choose oil-free sunscreen lotions, sprays, or gels.

One final word about sun protection: anytime you protect your skin, you should protect your eyes with sunglasses. The sun puts you as much at risk for cataracts as it does for skin cancers and premature aging.

Eat for Beauty

When I was a dermatology resident, the party line was that your diet did not affect your skin. One of my professors was fond of saying that the only way what you ate could give you acne was if you applied the grease from your pepperoni pizza to your face.

More than 10 years later, patients often hear the same thing. Read most dermatology textbooks, and you'll get a detailed analysis of the oil overproduction and bacterial overgrowth that characterize acne, but no mention of diet. You'll find comprehensive discussions of acne treatment, up to and including the most invasive and aggressive therapies currently available. But there's precious little about dietary modification, which is noninvasive and has no side effects. And what there is tends to be rather dismissive, such as this statement from a textbook entitled, *Acne and Rosacea* and devoted entirely to these skin conditions: "In summary, dietary regimens do not influence the course of the disease [acne]. This should be clearly stated to the patient."

These days, the lay press abounds with advice on what to eat to stay young and healthy. But patients still hear little of this from their dermatologists. I'm not surprised at the dearth of dietary advice in textbooks and from many doctors. After all, it's difficult to conduct a watertight scientific trial to prove the effects of your diet on your skin. And, as I discussed earlier, it's understandably difficult for many physicians to admit—to themselves, let alone to their patients—that medicine is not all neatly boxed logical science but contains large doses of fuzzy, empirical art. But I'm heartened by one recent acne study, albeit small, which questions the old dogma and supports what many of us have learned from experience and what I've told my patients for years: how we eat *does* significantly affect how we look. I hope this study will help physicians to feel a little more comfortable in dispensing vital dietary advice to all their patients, not just those with acne.

I'm a vegetarian. I'm not recommending you become one unless this really appeals to you. But please seriously consider increasing the fruits, grains, and vegetables in your diet and decreasing the meat and animal fats. Doing so is likely to prolong your life, prolong your beauty, and clear your acne. The key to changing your diet is moderation, not deprivation. You're much likelier to stick to a skin-healthy diet if it doesn't make you miserable.

A low-fat diet rich in grains, fruits, and vegetables increases your body's capacity to destroy free radicals. Put that together with the fact that this type of diet also seems to reduce skin cancers and precancers, and you've got to wonder how your diet affects other factors that depend on your free radical levels, like your rate of aging.

I believe there is a spiritual argument for reducing or eliminating meat from your diet too. Avoidance of meat can be a daily reaffirmation of the principles of nonviolence and compassion that characterize inner beauty.

What about dairy products? Many of my patients wonder about

their impact on the skin. "You have the skin of someone who doesn't drink milk!" one patient, Pauline, exclaimed to me a few years ago.

I was rather taken aback and only really pondered Pauline's words that evening as I brushed my teeth in front of the bathroom mirror. I had recently admitted to myself what I'd been in denial about for 5 years: I was lactose intolerant. I had not drunk milk in about 3 months. And, truth to tell, my skin *did* look better.

I'm not suggesting that you purge your fridge of dairy products tomorrow morning. Even I drink milk now, of the lactose-free variety. It's an important source of protein, calcium, and vitamins, especially if you're vegetarian or nearly so. I also eat yogurt at least twice a day. But Pauline's words reinforced what I had already learned from my experiences with my patients: to deny the impact of diet on skin is to deny common knowledge and common sense.

Take, for example, my patient Sumati, a software engineer who had emigrated from India, where she had eaten a largely dairy and vegetarian diet, with small portions of meat about once a week. Within a few months of arriving in Virginia, she was in my office with severe comedonal acne, the medical term for blackheads and whiteheads. Her previous dermatologist had attributed the breakout to the stress of changing countries. But when I spoke to Sumati, it was obvious that far from her being under tension due to her move, she relished it. Her new job was really not much of a change from her previous one in India. What had changed, however, was her diet. She'd happily adopted the customs of her new home and was eating meat twice a day.

Sumati was planning to become pregnant, so I was limited in how I could treat her. I recommended a glycolic acid cleanser, which would help with the acne and the resultant discolorations on her cheeks. And I wrote her a prescription for erythromycin gel, an antibiotic that's considered safe even when applied to the skin during pregnancy.

In the end, Sumati decided that she didn't want to use any medications while trying to get pregnant, an approach I fully supported. She did, however, take my advice to cut back on her consumption of red meat and animal fats. The results were dramatic. Her acne and her skin texture began to improve within a few weeks, and her skin was almost clear by the time she announced her pregnancy 6 months later.

I can give you many similar examples demonstrating the impact that diet has upon the skin. One of the most dramatic was my children's nanny. Within 4 months of walking into our house and adopting a low-fat vegetarian diet on weekdays, her acne cleared completely, to be replaced by a radiant glow—without any medical intervention whatsoever from me.

You'll note that I say "low-fat" and not "fat-free". The vogue for obsessively counting fat grams in your food may have passed, but I still meet patients like Jean, a writer in her mid-forties, who came to see me complaining of cracking skin and brittle nails.

"I don't understand it," she told me plaintively, "I drink loads of water, but I still have alligator skin!"

Your skin certainly needs water to function normally. And you'll look younger if you're well-hydrated, because wrinkles, facial gauntness and under-eye hollows are less apparent. Many of us get dehydrated from the low humidity of overheated or over-air conditioned offices and homes; an effect which is often compounded by busy schedules which leave us with little time to "think and drink"; that is, to listen to and to obey our bodies' thirst signals. However, Jean's dry skin and nails were due not to a lack of water, but to a lack of oil. When I questioned her about her lifestyle, it soon became apparent that she subscribed to the "zero fat" school of philosophy, in her quest to reduce her risk of heart disease. A rundown of her typical meals revealed an average fat intake of less than a teaspoon, or 5 grams, per day.

You may have heard how important "essential fatty acids" (EFA) are for your health. Nowhere is this truer than in your skin which, like the rest of your body, cannot live without these nutrients. What's more, EFA cannot be manufactured by your body; you must take sufficient quantities of them in your food or supplements. Recent research has fueled concerns that the typical American diet leaves you lacking in one of the two types of EFA—this is omega-3 EFA, which is also known as alpha-linolenic acid. Jean's fat restriction was short-changing her of EFA . . . and preventing her from achieving the good health she sought. Her problem skin and nails improved dramatically after she followed my advice to add some fat to her diet, in the form of omega-3 rich canola oil, nuts and fish.

The bottom line is, dietary modification is one skin regimen worth trying, primarily because it won't do you any harm and it may well do some good. Try changing how you eat for 6 months, and be your own judge. Remember that you are in the best position to determine what makes a difference for your skin—you know it better that anyone else, and you see it more often. If you think chocolate is flaring your acne or too much meat is dulling your skin, you're probably right, no matter what the experts say.

Sleep for Beauty

A consistent pattern of sleep is essential for beauty, and not just because it is a prerequisite for stress reduction. Sleep is the time during which your body—including your skin—restores and repairs itself. Studies show that even one night of sleep deprivation is enough to interfere with your skin's metabolism, impairing its functions as a protective barrier and its critical role in maintaining body temperature. Your skin is assaulted on a daily basis by the sun, potential infections and injuries, and many other invaders. Give it the time it needs to recoup.

Melissa was accustomed to burning the candle at both ends. By day, she ran a popular women's boutique with her best friend from college. And at night, she would hit the town with her crowd, often wearing one of her boutique's latest offerings. With her poise and statuesque physique, she was her own best model. Her evenings of clubbing gained her many customers, who would approach her to ask where she got her fabulous outfits and receive her business card in response.

Melissa cruised through her twenties footloose and fancy-free. But one day, shortly before her 30th birthday, she was shocked to notice a faint but distinct frown line between her eyebrows.

"It's unbearably depressing," she declared, prodding the offending wrinkle aggressively. "And it has to go."

Off it went, with a small dose of Botox. But as I surveyed Melissa's face, I knew it would be only a matter of time before another demon emerged to plague her. Just one look at her told me she was chronically sleep-deprived. The dark hollows under her eyes might give her a fashionably waiflike look right now, but in a few years, they would have developed into fully fledged bags as her stressed-out skin lost its elasticity.

It took a lot of persuasion for Melissa to stop burning the midnight oil. She insisted initially that it was essential to her boutique that she be out and about by night, displaying her wares. But when she returned for a maintenance Botox treatment 4 months later and I pointed out that her under-eye shadows had worsened even in that short time period, she began to see my point.

"I guess you're right," she sighed. "I can't live at 30 the way I did when I was 20."

Happily, Melissa's business did not suffer when she changed her frenetic lifestyle. And the improvement in her skin 6 months later told us both that she'd made the right decision.

There's another way in which sleep can affect how you look. Do you doze off with your face crushed into your pillow? If so, you may find yourself developing "sleep lines"—wrinkles which form as a direct result of habitual skin creasing. You can often identify these wrinkles by their peculiar orientation. Age-related wrinkles, such as those on your forehead or around your eyes, tend to follow the pull of gravity or underlying muscles, whereas sleep lines don't. They may lie horizontally along one cheek, diagonally across your chin . . . or in any direction which reflects the way your skin is creased as you sleep. I've had some success treating these lines with chemical peels or with collagen injections, but prevention is the best solution. If you can avoid the sleeping position that causes these lines, they will usually improve or even disappear with time.

Drink for Beauty

Studies show that alcoholic drinks and caffeine predispose you to free radical overload. As it breaks down in the body, alcohol directly generates free radicals. Alcohol also affects the other side of the equation, as does caffeine, by reducing your pineal gland's secretion of melatonin. As you may recall from earlier in this chapter, melatonin is a major part of your body's antioxidant system.

But what about the assertion that wine—red wine in particular—is good for you because it fights free radicals? In the lab, extracts of red or white wine do indeed have the potential to act as antioxidants. However, you may be surprised—and disappointed—to learn that what happens in the test tube does not seem to happen in real life. Drinking wine—or any other alcoholic beverage—has never been shown to increase the activity of anybody's antioxidant system.

The inner beauty rationale for reducing or eliminating alcohol or caffeine from your diet is similar to that for smoking: Even if you're not truly addicted, both alcohol and caffeine can serve as emotional crutches. Keep in mind also that they dehydrate you and may disturb your sleep patterns. Both of these effects can harm your outer beauty. Practice moderation, rather than deprivation, in regard to your alcohol and caffeine consumption.

A furor of speculation has swirled of late around tea, especially green tea. The jury is still out on whether green tea is an elixir of youth or a storm in a teacup. Some evidence strongly suggests that extracts of green tea containing complex molecules called polyphenols have powerful antioxidant capabilities. I've certainly found green tea extracts applied to the skin to be useful for many of my patients. For now, I'd encourage you to continue drinking green tea if you like it, but to consider the decaffeinated variety so that any potential benefits of the polyphenols you're imbibing are not offset by the caffeine you also take in. Consider substituting a decaffeinated variety for some or all of your daily coffee or regular tea.

Both Sumati, the engineer, and Melissa, the nightclubber, found that cutting back on their copious coffee drinking helped them sleep better, feel less stressed, and, ultimately, look more beautiful.

Get the Stress Out

I find it fascinating to think of the myriad of ways in which stress—whether outer or inner—telegraphs itself almost instantly to the skin. The reactions are so individual: you may break out with acne, I may suffer from mouth ulcers, and someone else may develop cold sores, eczema, or hair loss. Premature aging definitely comes high on everyone's list; we've all seen the drastic impact that stress has upon the youthful features of both the private and public figures in our lives.

There is solid scientific evidence that outer, physiological stress like sleep deprivation or extreme exertion can overload you with free radicals. I define inner, psychological stress as anything that perturbs your inner self. This includes anxiety, depression, and a host of other negative emotions. In midlife, your hormones may be in turmoil or, at the very least, a little shaken and stirred. You may find all varieties of stress peaking as you face the unique challenges of balancing your multifaceted life. As my patient Claire, whose mid-forties were marked by daily duels between her inner soccer mom and her outer career woman, put it, "I feel like a circus performer who's lost count of how many plates she's spinning!"

Scientific research reveals the intimate relationship between exercise and stress. Aerobic exercise reduces your physical response to stress; you tend to panic less or feel less anxious if you've exercised before you're put under stress, or even under the threat of stress. And regular exercise reduces fatigue and psychological distress in cancer patients undergoing chemotherapy. If you think regular exercise puts you in a better mood, you're right. Study subjects report a global improvement in their mood after an exercise session. They specifically cite decreases in tension, depression, fatigue and anger and an increase in feelings of vigor.

At least some benefits of exercise are due to increases in your blood levels of endorphins and enkephalins. Your body manufactures these natural, narcotic-like painkillers itself and they give you a heightened sense of well-being, even euphoria. The intensely pleasurable surges of endorphins and enkephalins can get you healthily "hooked" on exercise. They also increase your tolerance to pain and stress. And they are part of a complex feedback loop that regulates your reproductive hormones and adrenaline levels.

I consider regular exercise to be an essential part of any beauty program. If you've not yet been able to motivate yourself to maintain a regular exercise routine, envision the beauty benefits: the enhanced blood flow to your skin, reduced stress, and the feelings of inner well-being. I can frequently spot, simply by her glow, a patient who works out seriously.

(However, it's worth noting that the relationship between exercise and free radicals is not clear-cut. The studies show that if you exercise too strenuously, you'll actually increase your free radical levels. It's not known yet if there's a certain threshold beyond which this occurs. By exercising regularly, you'll strengthen your body's antioxidant system, which can defend you from the extra free radicals you produce.)

Internal stress is detrimental to inner beauty. You cannot focus on the development and projection of your inner beauty if your mind is clouded with unsettling thoughts. Nor can you sleep regularly and well, a prerequisite for beauty.

Intuitively, every woman knows that stress affects how she looks. This connection is generally insidious but occasionally dramatic, as in the case of Marie Antoinette, the queen whose hair was said to have turned white overnight during the French Revolution—probably the result of her suddenly shedding all her dark hair due to alopecia areata, a stress-related type of hair loss.

I spoke before of the benefits of meditation, which promotes physical relaxation and mental peace. Some of the well-established medical benefits of meditation—reduced stress, improved blood circulation, and reduced anxiety and depression—are tremendously important in the context of beauty.

You can begin your stress management by adopting regular sleeping, eating and exercise habits. Add meditation, and you may be amazed at the results. Even if you're only relieved of outside distractions for 5 or 10 minutes a day, the resultant stress reduction lasts far longer and can truly transform your life.

Hormonal Balance for Beauty

Around the time during my training that I realized dermatology was my calling, I stumbled upon a television program about Hollywood film studios in the first half of the last century and the all-powerful control they exerted over their stars. I was fascinated to learn that one studio even kept precise records of its actresses' menstrual cycles, the better to optimize makeup and lighting as their skin changed with their monthly hormone shifts.

As bizarre and "Big Brotherly" as this practice may seem, there is some rationale behind it. Your skin does indeed cycle under the influence of your hormones, not just in how acne-prone it is—an effect all too familiar to many women—but also in its texture and pigmentation. For instance, at the time of ovulation, your skin signals your fecundity loud and clear, yet subliminally to the psyche of every passerby, by significantly lightening in color.

You'll recall that lighter skin is theorized to be an evolutionary hallmark of beauty because it shows the flushing of sexual excitement—and receptivity—more readily; think of Snow White with her pale skin and rosy cheeks. This is another powerful example of how beauty, sex and fertility are inextricably entwined. Your beauty (by evolutionary criteria, at any rate), your ability to display sexual responsiveness and your fertility peak at precisely the same moment.

As you age, and the function of your ovaries begins to decline, there are complex changes in the balance between the female hormones estrogen and progesterone. Your levels of estrogen ultimately decrease at an individual rate as you approach menopause. This has profound and permanent effects upon your skin because estrogen and progesterone are needed for the efficient production of healthy collagen. Skin aging seems to accelerate during perimenopause and menopause, but we won't fully understand the reasons for this until we have a clearer picture of the ways that hormones affect our skin. Many women are dismayed to find that their skin becomes noticeably drier and more wrinkled as they enter midlife. My patient Lisa, noticing her suddenly deepening crow's-feet and smile lines, told me eloquently, "Since I hit 35, my face has been falling apart."

If you experience premature menopause by the age of forty or so, or "medical menopause" because your ovaries are removed or damaged, the impact on your skin—as on the rest of your body—tends to be more dramatic. This is presumed to be because your estrogen-progesterone balance is disrupted suddenly, rather than shifting gradually as it does with natural menopause. What's interesting is that many women report significant changes in their skin even if their ovaries are preserved after hysterectomy. For instance, Ivy, a forty-year-old homemaker, noticed a sudden increase in wrinkles and skin looseness around her jawline and eyes within a year of a hysterectomy which removed part of her uterus but left both her ovaries intact. I could see these changes, too. The traditional medical understanding of hysterectomy is that removal of the uterus alone stops your menstrual periods but does not affect the functioning of your ovaries or your hormonal balance. Many women can attest to the fact that this may be an over-simplification. Ivy also noticed that her cyclical symptoms of breast tenderness and moodiness worsened after her hysterectomy.

A few years ago, women complaining of symptoms such as Ivy's were often exhorted to take hormone therapy, which contains estrogen and usually progesterone too. The women who swear that hormone therapy keeps them young are partially right. Studies show that supplementary hormones can prevent skin dryness and wrinkling. But the days when Hollywood movie stars and everyday women alike touted hormone therapy as the secret of youthful skin are over. In light of recent research that suggests that it may actually be dangerous, at least for some women, hormone therapy has become a mixed blessing. The same may be true of soy, which contains natural, plant-derived estrogens and has recently become the mainstay of many a woman's midlife health and beauty plan. Some dietary supplements contain doses of soy which greatly exceed what you'd take in naturally by eating a well-balanced diet that includes some tofu or other soy-containing foods.

Women—and their physicians—are faced with more complexities than ever before when deciding whether or not they should take hormone therapy. Of course, there may be good medical reasons for you to take hormones before, during, or after menopause . . . at least, for a defined time period. But keeping your skin young is not one of them, especially in light of new studies suggesting that the potentially serious risks of hormone therapy may outweigh the health benefits for many women. Whether or not you take hormones is an individual decision for you and your health care professional to make together, in the context of your overall health. But the long term effects of this therapy are too uncertain for your skin to ever factor into this picture. There are so many other, less controversial lifestyle options which are proven to benefit your skin, without exposing you to potential health risks.

Consider this too: the term "hormone replacement" is really a misleading misnomer. The declining levels of female hormones that you experience as you pass through perimenopause are natural, as is menopause itself. Menopause is as much a part of a woman's life as the hormonal surges of puberty and the years of monthly menstrual cycles.

Hormone therapy *is* replacement for a woman who's had her ovaries removed before menopause. But it's actually *supplementation* that modifies the natural hormone levels of a woman who has her ovaries and is in, or approaching, menopause.

We deny this essential truth when we label the estrogen and progesterone pills we pop as "replacement," rather than the supplementation they are. And we also do ourselves a disservice by buying into the insidious concept that menopause is a disease or deficiency that must be managed with "replacement therapy."

Let's be honest with ourselves and see hormone therapy for what it is. And let's view menopause in the light of our new understanding and knowledge: as an important life passage with the potential to empower and uplift us in spirit and body. Because then we can allow ourselves to walk in beauty at *every* stage of life.

chapter nine

Lotions, Potions, and Pills—What You Can Do at Home

Everything should be made as simple as possible, but not simpler.

—Albert Einstein

"Here it all is—I emptied out my bathroom cabinet!" exclaimed Charlotte, a 36-year-old advertising consultant as she breezed into the exam room.

I generally encourage my new patients to review all their current skin care products with me. This starting point helps us devise an effective and simple skin care regimen. I can also identify any products that might be causing skin reactions or are otherwise unsuitable for my patients' faces. Charlotte had followed my advice quite literally, and now she was panting slightly as she heaved three substantial, very full shopping bags onto the exam table. When I opened the first one, a cornucopia of bottles spilled out and even I felt momentarily overwhelmed.

The bulging bags and cosmetic purses that Charlotte and her comrades bring into my office might tempt you into thinking that these women are to skin care what Imelda Marcos was to shoes. But the problem here is not just excessive spending. Consider, too, the wasted hours, even if each product purchase took just 15 minutes. Why would any busy woman in her right mind willingly fritter away the little spare time she has listening to sales pitch after sales pitch at cosmetic counters? I think the answer has more to do with bewilderment than self-indulgence.

During my dermatology residency in Chicago, one of my fellow trainees told me laughingly how she and her father—a dermatologist too—used to visit department store cosmetic counters together for kicks. They'd go incognito and get days of entertainment from the bizarre skin care advice they received. I vividly remember visiting one of those counters myself at a dermatology conference several years ago, accompanied by a friend who reported that "these people can custom-blend makeup to match any skin." The white-coated woman took one look at my face, made a few perfunctory attempts to find something on her shelves, and then told me, "This isn't going to work because you have too much olive in your skin."

This type of experience may be highly amusing—or at worst mildly irritating—for me and for my professional colleagues. After all, our forays into department store beauty carry no emotional investment whatsoever. But it's hardly fun for you if you're sold the dream of an effortlessly perfect complexion by cosmetics counters and beauty ads and end up in a nightmare where your bathroom cabinet is full of pricey products and your skin is still no better.

Flip through a women's magazine or two, cruise the local department stores, tune in to the latest television infomercial, and you may begin to agree with H. G. Wells that advertising is legalized lying. Beauty ads are a genre unto themselves. Even as they push our consumer buttons, they also push the envelope where veracity is concerned.

Strictly speaking, the statements made in these ads are not inaccurate. But what they imply is often beyond outrageous. Take "reduces the appearance of wrinkles," for instance—a tantalizing promise whose appeal to the unsuspecting is belied by the fact that you can reduce the *appearance* of your wrinkles even by rubbing Crisco into your face. Or consider concoctions whose names contain weasel words like "lift," "peel," and "surge" to imbue them instantly with the aura of cosmetic surgery.

Then there's the wide variation in prices. What exactly are you paying for? Deceptive packaging can make a few teaspoons of cream look like twice the volume. Most of all, what do the women portrayed in the ads have to do with you? Even the "mature" ones are airbrushed within an inch of their lives; wrinkles are apparently unacceptable even in a wrinkle ad. Confusion reigns supreme for many women where lotions and potions are concerned. Charlotte, surveying the debris of her quest for good skin, put it succinctly: "I've spent over $800 on this stuff, and I've no idea what it's all for!"

Take heart; there *are* good skin care products out there. The challenge is to sort the wheat from the chaff. And that's what I'm going to help you to do. You'll also learn how to choose the right skin care advisor—someone who has insight into what will really work for you. I'll end this chapter with my 7-Minute Amazing Skin Regimen for several skin types (page 173). But first a few general principles about products.

Make 30 your ceiling. Think carefully about purchasing any over-the-counter skin care product that costs more than $30. Products that require a prescription or must be dispensed from a doctor's office are generally more potent. For example, over-the-counter face creams tend to have a lower concentration of glycolic acid than their physician-dispensed cousins. I think a product containing less of an active ingredient should cost less too.

Avoid expensive "window dressing." The upscale (and costly) perfumes in some creams or makeup offer you no benefits and may actually give you a rash. The same is true of some natural botanical extracts. Be skeptical of beguilingly-named wonder ingredients that probably can't do anything, scientifically speaking, because all they do is to sit on your skin's surface.

Aim for simplicity. Your chances of achieving good skin are *not* directly proportional to the amount of time and money you spend or the number of items you use. Department store beauty counters—and even physicians' offices—often attempt to sell you a whole "system" when a few well-chosen products will do just as well.

Don't believe all the hype. A word of caution about books, magazines, and advertisements that tempt you with the promise of wrinkle improvement from an at-home skin regimen in just a few days. If you understand the structure of your skin and the length of the cycles it goes through, you'll understand that it's nonsense for anyone—whether a physician or an advertiser—to claim that skin aging can be reversed by their skin products in such a short period of time. Sure, one or two applications of a cream that hydrates your skin will make it feel tighter, and one that exfoliates it will make it look and feel smoother. But it takes weeks or months for a cream to increase collagen production in your dermis or to thicken your epidermis, to give you true reversal of aging.

Believe this: at-home skin care is definitely worth the bother. You can achieve an enormous amount with the right regimen—and also optimize your results from cosmetic procedures, should you decide to go that route. As I constantly stress to my patients, successful at-home skin rejuvenation is all about consistency and patience. If you use effective products and stick with them, you *will* see results.

One final note: some of the studies on products that I refer to were conducted or sponsored by the companies that make the products. That doesn't mean that these studies are not valid. But it does mean that as with the rest of this book, you should supplement the information here with what your own physician tells you so that you get a complete picture of your skin care options.

I mention some of the brand-name products that I dispense from my office to my patients and some that I use myself. While I have consulted for some of the manufacturers of these brands, that doesn't mean that I'm endorsing them above other products on the market, many of which may be equally good. My criteria for mentioning a product are that it gives my patients results beyond what they can achieve from drugstore or salon products and that it's cost-effective. I don't recommend "big-name" products unless it's the results that are big and not merely the prices.

Moisturizers: Let Yourself Shine a Little

Look at a child to see how your skin was meant to be: it glows with moisture. Children don't worry about oil, nor do they powder their noses into submission. What's interesting to me is the ferocity many of my patients display toward their shiny skin. My patient Audrey complained that her face was too oily. Yet I saw dryness instead on her cheeks and around her eyes. Audrey described her skin as "disgusting" and buried her offending nose in her hands, too ashamed to let me see it. Other patients tell me their skin is "gross" or "horrible."

What is the cause of this "oil phobia"? Personally, I think it's a reflection of our fear of bodily secretions in general. As women, we are taught from an early age that there's very little our bodies secrete that is desirable. Look at what we do to ourselves under the guise of feminine hygiene—the name itself a clear implication that *not* to do so is to be unfeminine or unhygienic. Zoologist Desmond Morris has noted the irony of women's scrubbing away their own natural body secretions, including pheromones, only to anoint themselves with the bodily secretions of other animals, in the form of perfumes and musks.

I'm not advocating that you skip your daily shower. But I do think it's important for you to understand the difference between clean skin and denuded skin. When your skin's natural protective oil barrier is removed, it's vulnerable to damage. And mysterious as pheromones may be, we do know that they play an important role—almost certainly larger than we'll ever appreciate—in nonverbal communication. You'll never know how purging yourself of your pheromones affects others' perceptions of your beauty.

The flip side of oil phobia is the wholesale faith in the curative powers of moisturizers. Moisturizing by itself can't make your wrinkles disappear, no matter what the "miracle creams" seem to promise. But moisturizers can make your wrinkles less noticeable by giving your skin a healthy, youthful glow that distracts the eye from your imperfections.

You have probably heard the oft-repeated exhortation to look for a moisturizer that's hypoallergenic and noncomedogenic. But what does this dermatological jargon really mean? A hypoallergenic cream is *less* likely to cause skin allergies, but it is not guaranteed to make your skin happy. I've personally reacted to a number of over-the-counter hypoallergenic creams. However, most skin reactions are due to fragrance, and hypoallergenic creams are by definition fragrance-free. In general, looking for a jar with "**hypoallergenic**" on the label is a good strategy—it lessens the odds of a reaction.

A **noncomedogenic** cream is supposed to not block up your skin pores and cause acne. Alternative terms you'll see on some products are "**nonacnegenic**" and "won't clog pores." But in fact there's controversy about the test a cream must pass to acquire any of these three labels. If the ingredients of the cream do not produce blackheads or whiteheads when they're applied to a rabbit's ear in the lab, the cream passes the test. Whether or not this test is directly relevant to human skin in the real world is the subject of some debate. I generally advise my patients to look for noncomedogenic products. But if there's one particular cream they're in love with and I don't feel it's causing a problem, I won't force a patient to switch, even if the "hypoallergenic, noncomedogenic" mantra is not on the jar.

Read the ingredients of most modern moisturizers, and you may feel you're back in science class. As one of my patients recently bemoaned, "Whatever happened to good old cold cream?" Well, good old cold cream is still around, but there are some good new ingredients too. **Hyaluronic acid** has powerful water-retaining properties and is a component of the substance that cements collagen and elastic fibers in your dermis together. When applied to your skin surface in a cream, it's very effective at holding in moisture and gives your skin a smooth, silky feel. **Glycerin** works in a similar way.

Some new ingredients are not so good, or at least not much use. For instance, **collagen**, **elastic**, and **epidermal growth factor** are found naturally within your skin and contribute to its youthful tightness and smoothness. However, there's no evidence whatsoever that applying them to your skin has any effect. These substances cannot penetrate to the layers of your skin where they might be effective; they simply sit on the surface.

You can get an idea of whether a moisturizer is right for you before you even open the jar, simply by looking at the ingredient list. A moisturizer is basically a combination of oil and water, and the proportion of each determines how it feels on your skin. Water is invariably the first ingredient. The higher up that oils feature on the ingredient list, the likelier the moisturizer is to be a heavier cream, rather than a lighter lotion. The lightest lotions are actually oil-free, and even the oiliest skin can benefit from the hydration they provide.

If you really dislike the weighty feel of a cream or lotion, try an oil-free moisturizing gel. And be prepared to change your moisturizer with the seasons. Many women—including me—find that they need a heavier moisturizer in winter, when the air is dry and cold, than in summer. Keep in mind also that what's perfect for a sweltering August afternoon in Washington, D.C., may leave your skin thirsty for more on a zero-humidity morning in Denver.

Cosmeceuticals: the Alphas, Betas, and Vitamin Cs of Beauty

Look up the term "**cosmeceutical**" in your dictionary, and it's likely you'll draw a blank. Yet the products found in this controversial group have almost certainly permeated your consciousness. Broadly speaking, a cosmeceutical is a product that lies somewhere between a pharmaceutical (a prescription medication) and a cosmetic. Some are available over-the-counter at your drugstore or at salons, and some are available at doctors' offices. All are nonprescription and, as such, not regulated by the FDA (Food and Drug Administration) in the same way that prescription medications are.

And that's where the controversy lies. Cosmeceuticals do not have to undergo the same stringent testing for effectiveness and safety that prescription drugs do. Some are no doubt exceedingly effective and very safe, and they often combine today's modern science with the wisdom of antiquity. The challenge is to find those that *do* work and avoid those that are just prettily packaged hype.

Once upon a time, this was simple: we had few cosmeceuticals besides **glycolic acid**. Now you may find yourself spoiled, and bewildered, by choice. You're bombarded with alpha hydroxy this, beta hydroxy that, and vitamins with every letter of the alphabet. So what works and what doesn't?

Alpha, Beta, and Poly Hydroxy Acids and Retinoids

As I mentioned earlier, **alpha hydroxy acids (AHAs)** have a venerable history. In their natural form, they are derived from sugars in milk—like the lactic acid in Cleopatra's sour milk baths. Today they are synthetically manufactured for purity and consistency of activity.

AHAs have been scientifically proven to act against many of the changes aging skin undergoes. They boost sluggish exfoliation by microscopically peeling away the dead skin cells at the top of your epidermis, to reveal the younger cells below. This gives you what I call the "glycolic glow," by preventing the buildup of dead cells that dull your skin's surface and by fading age spots and other discolorations. This exfoliation can also help acne, by unblocking clogged pores.

AHAs also thicken your epidermis, reversing (to some extent) the thinning that occurs with age. In addition, they're extremely efficient at increasing your skin's ability to attract and retain moisture. Their hydrating effect is far more powerful than you can achieve with a regular moisturizer, and this is why AHAs make your skin feel smooth and firm. Perhaps most exciting of all is the possibility that AHAs may not only improve the effects of aging but also directly attack the root cause of aging, by destroying free radicals in your skin.

The beauty industry holds conflicting views over which member of the AHA family is most effective. Many manufacturers prefer **glycolic acid**, feeling that it's the most effective AHA because its small molecule penetrates your epidermis easily. Others tout the benefits of **lactic acid**, malic acid, or other AHAs with larger molecules, on the grounds that they may be less irritating to your skin.

There's also some debate about whether the acidity, or pH, of your AHA cream makes any difference. AHAs are naturally quite acidic, but some manufacturers reduce this acidity by adding other chemicals, with the aim of making them gentler on your skin. The question is whether this process, known as buffering, also makes AHAs less effective. The terms you may see on your jar of cream are "unbuffered," which means the AHA is in its naturally acidic state and has a low pH, or "partially buffered," which means the AHA has been made less acidic and has a higher pH. I personally prefer AHA creams that are unbuffered or only slightly buffered as I've found them to be more effective. The glycolic acid products I recommend in my office, and use intermittently myself, are from the Topix (Dermatopix), Glyderm, and Glytone lines.

In general, my patients don't have many problems with skin irritation from AHAs because my strategy is to recommend them only for patients I feel are likely to tolerate them. I turn to less irritating cosmeceuticals like **antioxidants** for patients who would be likely to experience stinging or burning with AHAs.

Beta hydroxy acids (BHAs) also rev up your skin's natural exfoliation processes by removing the uppermost dead cells of your epidermis. The main BHA used in skin creams is **salicylic acid**, which is related to aspirin. BHAs have the potential to calm skin inflammation, and because of this, your skin may be able to tolerate them even if it's sensitive to AHAs. This anti-inflammatory effect may also be one of the reasons they're so useful in treating acne, which typically involves skin inflammation. I tend to use BHAs for patients with acne, including blackheads and whiteheads.

Poly hydroxy acids (PHAs), like BHAs, also exfoliate your skin and are a better choice for sensitive skin than AHAs. The most commonly used PHA is **gluconolactone**. This PHA may appear on its own or be combined with AHAs, with the aim of reducing skin irritation.

Retinoids are a family of skin rejuvenators derived from the antioxidant, vitamin A. The family includes **retinol**, which is an over-the-counter form of vitamin A; and **tretinoin** and **tazarotene**, which are vitamin A derivatives available by prescription. Tretinoin cream and gel are marketed under the brand names Renova, Retin-A, and Avita. Tazarotene goes by the brand names Avage and Tazorac. Because these are prescription medications, they are not truly cosmeceuticals. But I'll discuss them here together with retinol and other vitamin A-derived creams available over-the-counter.

Renova, which consists of tretinoin in a moisturizing cream base, is available in two strengths. It is specifically marketed as an anti-aging treatment and is approved by the FDA for this purpose. It works by fighting many of the aging processes going on in your skin. Studies show that it improves sun-aged skin, by making it smoother and more elastic and by reducing fine wrinkles, discolorations, and precancerous skin growths. Renova works by making your epidermis more efficient at producing new skin cells and exfoliating old ones; it also boosts the ability of your dermis to produce new collagen and elastic. These studies have not been done with Retin-A or Avita because they are marketed as acne treatments. However, they do contain the same active ingredient as Renova, in various strengths.

Where Retin-A and Avita differ from Renova is in their base—that is, the rest of the product besides the active ingredient, tretinoin—and exactly how the tretinoin is formulated. Both Avita and Retin-A come as creams or gels. I find that Avita is a little less drying than Retin-A.

Avage is the newest retinoid in the anti-aging armory. Its active ingredient is tazarotene. Studies show that Avage has similar effects to Renova, decreasing fine wrinkles and skin discolorations. Tazarotene is also marketed as Tazorac, which is used to treat psoriasis, but has not been approved by the FDA for the treatment of aging skin.

Retinol is an effective over-the-counter option in fighting skin damage from free radicals. However, it's not as effective as its prescription-only cousins because it does not penetrate your skin as well and is not as active even when it has penetrated.

I usually prescribe or recommend retinoids for use at night because they are inactivated by sunlight. They also make your skin more sensitive to the sun. If you use retinoids, it's doubly important that you protect yourself from the sun during the day even if you're using them at night: first, to prevent reactions due to your increased sun sensitivity, and second, so that the anti-aging effect of your retinoid is not negated by the aging effects of the sun.

The Red Test

The anti-aging therapies I've just discussed—AHAs, BHAs, PHAs, and retinoids—are highly effective and the mainstay of many of my patients' regimens. But, as I'm fond of telling my patients, they must be used on the right skin and by the right hands. My Red Test tells you whether or not you have the right skin. Do you tend to get facial redness when your skin is dry, when you're overheated or overchilled, when you exert yourself, or just any time for no apparent reason? If so, I wouldn't recommend any of the above treatments—with the exception of over-the-counter retinol and perhaps PHAs, no matter how effective they are—because they'll only make you redder. You may have rosacea, a form of adult acne that I've mentioned before and will discuss later in this chapter. In my terms, you have the wrong skin for most of these products, which I think of as Red Flamers.

Tretinoin and tazarotene stimulate the formation of new blood vessels in the dermis of your skin. The increased blood vessels often make your skin a little pinker, giving you a rosy glow. You may recall that these blood vessels feed your epidermis with vital nutrients and remove waste products. You may also recall that as your skin ages, the number of blood vessels decreases, which causes your epidermis to function less well. So as tretinoin and tazarotene counteract this decrease, they have a beneficial anti-aging effect.

But if your face already tends to be red, Renova, Retin-A, Avita or Avage may well leave you looking like a tomato, rather than a rose. And there's another reason that retinoids, as well as alpha and beta hydroxy acids, may make you red—they can inflame your skin.

That's where the right hands come in. I believe it's essential that you take your skin to someone who not only understands it but also understands how to select from the full range of options that are available for improving your skin. If you go to a cosmetic counter, salon, or doctor that is familiar with only glycolic acid or vitamin A, then that's all you're going to get, regardless of whether or not it's the right choice for your skin. I see the unhappy results of this cookie-cutter dispensing all the time.

Estelle frequently visited her ophthalmologist because she needed regular checkups for the raised pressure in her eyes, a condition known as glaucoma. On one visit, she noticed in the waiting room some new signs advertising skin care products and vitamins. When she inquired at the front desk, she was told that a physician assistant, who specialized in skin care and nutrition and was supervised by the eye doctor, had joined the practice. Estelle was intrigued and immediately booked an appointment for a skin consultation. She had just turned 50 and was becoming increasingly aware of changes in her skin as she approached menopause. One-stop shopping for her eyes and her skin sounded like a great idea.

Estelle didn't see her doctor at all during her visit. She later learned that the physician assistant performed skin consultations on the days when the doctor was out of his office, doing surgery in the hospital. Thus, he was never in the office to directly supervise the assistant. Estelle left the consultation with more than $100 worth of products, including a glycolic acid cleanser, toner, facial cream, and eye cream.

When she came to see me a week later, her face was red, burning, and peeling. Worse, the eye cream had inflamed her eyelids so much that she was having difficulty inserting the eyedrops she needed for her glaucoma.

Once I had cleared up Estelle's reaction to the glycolic acid and her skin had returned to normal, I was able to rejuvenate her skin very effectively, and with no skin irritation, by selecting from the next group of cosmeceuticals I'll discuss. I think of them as Red Tamers that not only rejuvenate skin but also tone down facial redness, rather than turn it up.

Antioxidants and Furfuryladenine: Tame Those Free Radicals

Think of antioxidants as being part of a one–two strategy, along with sun protection. You can (and should) protect yourself from excess sun exposure with clothing and sunscreen and by limiting your time outdoors during high-sun periods. But despite all this, some sun is going to get through to your skin. That's where antioxidants can help, by mopping up the resultant free radicals. Of course, they'll be effective against free radicals from any source, not just the sun. (I generally recommend using antioxidants in the morning so that they will protect you throughout the day.)

Like vitamin A and its derivatives, **vitamin C** is an antioxidant that works against free radicals in your skin. This powerful vitamin also stimulates your dermis to produce more collagen, making your skin smoother and tighter. I've also found vitamin C cream very effective for decreasing facial redness and fading brown age spots and discolorations.

In studies, an active vitamin C concentration of at least 5 percent was needed for these anti-aging effects. Unfortunately, vitamin C is unstable and breaks down easily; if it's exposed to oxygen in the air, it loses its effectiveness entirely. Many of the most heavily advertised and popular vitamin C preparations suffer from this problem of stability. They are often packaged in brown bottles to protect them from sun exposure. Of course, an ordinary white plastic jar would do the same. But these brown bottles conveniently disguise the fact that the product has itself turned brown due to the breakdown of vitamin C. Topix Pharmaceuticals makes a stabilized vitamin C cream or serum called Citrix, which I've found to be quite effective and relatively nonirritating to my patients' skin.

Copper peptide and **coenzyme Q_{10}** are two antioxidants that have the potential to fight free radical damage. Some studies show that copper peptide is a highly potent stimulator of collagen production in the dermis—perhaps even more so than retinoids or vitamin C. I use copper peptide creams made by ProCyte, particularly Neova eye cream and milk cleanser, in my skin care regimens for patients who cannot tolerate AHAs.

The newest products to enter the antioxidant arena contain **green tea extracts of polyphenols**. Replenix cream or serum, made by Topix Pharmaceuticals, is the mainstay of many of my Red Tamer regimens. I've found that it makes skin smoother and more lustrous, decreases facial redness, and fades discolorations.

Kinerase is not an antioxidant, but I include it in my armory of Red Tamers. Manufactured by ICN Pharmaceuticals, it contains a plant-derived anti-withering agent called **furfuryladenine**. Amazingly, what works in plants also seems to work in human skin. Like retinoids, Kinerase seems to make skin smoother and reduce wrinkles and discolorations. But unlike retinoids, it is nonirritating and does not make you more sensitive to the sun. Furfuryladenine is also available under the name, Kinetin.

In Estelle's case, I recommended Neova cleanser and eye cream, which contain copper peptide, for twice-daily use. She applies Replenix cream, which contains green tea polyphenol extract, to her face and neck every morning, followed by an oil-free sunscreen. And she applies Kinerase cream every night. Her natural facial redness and her age spots have improved so dramatically that she has claimed to be "in love" with these products.

Vitamin E

Vitamin E is also an antioxidant, and some people swear by it for healing. Have you heard of people breaking open vitamin E capsules intended to be taken by mouth and rubbing the oil into their skin injuries or scars? In fact, there's no evidence that doing so improves skin healing or scars, other than by moisturizing them. Plus, there's a good chance you may be allergic to vitamin E applied to your skin. Nevertheless, vitamin E is added to a number of over-the-counter skin creams. If you use one of these and develop facial redness or itching, be attuned to the fact that you may be reacting to vitamin E.

Other Vitamins

Some skin creams contain vitamins that are not antioxidants, such as the **B vitamins, biotin, niacin**, and **riboflavin**. These vitamins are naturally present in your skin and needed for its regular functions, but it's not clear what they do when applied in cream form. **Yeast extract**, which appears on some ingredient lists, is rich in B vitamins.

In your body, **vitamin K** is needed for your blood to clot normally, and it's sometimes added to creams with the aim of decreasing bruising or spider veins. While I've not found vitamin K to have any effect on spider veins, it does seem to decrease bruising and even dark under-eye circles in some of my patients (although the scientific basis for these effects is not clear).

Masks: The Pause That Refreshes, Body and Soul

A mask is not strictly necessary for great skin. But it can be a wonderful uplifter used either at home or in the office. I recommend two types of mask to my patients. One is a **clay mint mask**, made by Topix pharmaceuticals, which gently removes excess oil from your pores. The other is a **hydrating mask**, made by Dermatologic Cosmetic Laboratories, which moisturizes dry skin. Both can be used at home one or more times a week.

If you like masks and have the time for them, then use them. At the very least, they're stress reducers. Do consult your physician to find a mask that's suitable for your skin type and that complements the rest of your skin care regimen.

Toners: Feel-Good Beauty

Strictly speaking, your skin doesn't really need a toner. Toners are touted for use after your cleanser, to remove dirt from your face and close your skin pores. In fact, most of the brown debris you see on your cotton ball after toning your face is not dirt but dead skin cells and traces of makeup that remain after you've used a cleanser. And nothing, not even a toner, can close your skin pores; skin pores cannot close. What toners will do is remove excess oil from your pores and give your skin a clean, fresh feeling.

If your skin doesn't feel "dressed" without a toner, go ahead and use one. Stay away from formulations that contain a lot of alcohol as these may irritate or dry your skin and even increase your chances of developing spider veins on your nose and cheeks. Toners with a little **witch hazel** or glycolic acid may work for you if you have oily or acne-prone skin. I use a Topix toner containing witch hazel and glycolic acid for facials in my office, and some patients like to use it at home too.

Bleaching Creams: Out, Out, Spots

Bleaching creams are used to fade age spots or sunspots and other skin discolorations. **Hydroquinone** is the active ingredient in the two creams I commonly prescribe, Glyquin and Claripel. I've found them to be very effective and to cause skin irritation only rarely. Over-the-counter fading creams contain about half as much hydroquinone that you'll find in the prescription creams, which makes them much less effective. Hydroquinone works by reducing your skin's production of melanin pigment.

Whichever bleaching cream you use, it will be only as effective as the sun protection you practice too. Otherwise, as fast as the cream does its thing, the sun will be stimulating your skin to produce more melanin. My patient Lenora used a generic hydroquinone cream for 6 months for the patchy facial discoloration she'd developed during her pregnancy. But she had no results other than an itching face until I switched her to Glyquin and advised her to wear sunscreen and avoid excessive sun exposure every day. Even I was stunned to see how clear her skin became after just 4 months.

One warning about bleaching creams. Creams containing more than 5 percent hydroquinone should be avoided at all costs as they can cause skin discoloration of a particularly dark and disfiguring type by triggering a process known as ochronosis. The resultant discoloration is virtually impossible to treat. Creams of this type are not available in the United States, but they have been sold in other countries, such as South Africa, where they're notorious for this terrible side effect.

Supplements: Do, But Don't Overdo

If you're taking care of yourself and eating well, you should be getting enough of the vitamins and other nutrients you need from your diet, including the free radical–destroying vitamins A, C, and E. There's no harm in supplementing what you eat with a one-a-day multivitamin. I take one because I don't eat meat and thus might be at risk for iron or vitamin B deficiency.

But there can be harm in overdoing your supplements. The supplements themselves may interact dangerously with other medications you're taking, or you may experience side effects from overdosing. Take vitamin E, for instance. It's blood thinning effect may be dangerous if you're already on other blood thinners like aspirin or coumadin. And controversy rages over whether taking vitamin E in capsule form even gives you the same benefits as naturally occurring vitamin E in foods.

Angela, a doctor's wife in her late forties, came to me in great distress because of hair loss. To an outside observer, her hair was still lush and full. But when she showed me pictures of herself taken 5 years previously, I could see what she meant. Her hair was indeed thinner, especially at her temples and crown. After consideration, I discussed with Angela the possibility that her thinning hair might be normal as she approached menopause. Her menstrual periods had been irregular for the preceding year or so, and she'd recently begun to experience mild, but definite, hot flashes. Her OB/GYN had run some hormonal blood tests that showed that her levels of estrogen and progesterone were beginning to decline.

What's more, she had a family history of hair loss; both her mother's father and her mother's uncle had gone bald in their forties. This type of hair loss, known as androgenetic alopecia, does tend to run more on your mother's side of the family. Unlike a man, a woman who inherits this type of hair loss does not tend to develop bald spots. Instead, she loses hair more diffusely, especially from the crown and sides of her scalp.

Even in a situation where I think I've identified why a woman's hair is thinning, I think it's important to investigate further to see whether there are any additional medical reasons. I often have to be a real detective to solve the mystery of hair loss. So I ran some blood tests to check for various causes of hair loss, including anemia and underactivity or overactivity of Angela's thyroid gland. These all came back negative.

As I was discussing these results with Angela, I reviewed her medical history again. She had told me during her previous visit that she was not taking any medications, vitamins or health food supplements. But when I asked her about medications again, it jogged her memory.

"You know what—I completely forgot this before, but I am taking some natural herbs to help with the symptoms of menopause," she told me.

When I saw the ingredients of the three herbal supplements Angela had been taking for more than a year, the mystery was solved. Each contained vitamin A. When taken together, they would overdose Angela with ten times the recommended daily amount. And hair loss is a typical symptom of vitamin A overdosage.

A full year after Angela stopped taking the supplements, her hair had finally become her crowning glory once again. In the meantime, I recommended that she use Tricomin shampoo and hair spray, which contain a copper peptide antioxidant. I've found that they reduce hair shedding in many of my patients and make the hair they have look much fuller and thicker.

We can learn two lessons from Angela's story. The first is that anyone—even a doctor's wife—can inadvertently overdose on vitamins and pay the price. The second is that anyone may benefit from being asked the same question more than once. My patients sometimes wonder why my assistant asks them the details of their medical history, and I then repeat some of the questions when I enter the room. I do this because I've found that it's the best way to ensure I have all the information I need to solve each patient's medical mystery.

Makeup: Less Is More

Remember the beauty book of my childhood? *101 Ways to Bring Out Your Beauty* summarized the state-of-the-art of 1970's beauty knowledge. If your lips were "too full," you were to cover them with concealer, draw a thinner line within them with lip liner, and then fill this in with lipstick. If your eyelids were "too shallow," you were to cover them with dark eye shadow to make them look deeper. The emphasis was on camouflaging your imperfections and conforming to an idealized, rigid standard of beauty.

And—oh, dear—remember the makeup of your youth? Blue mascara and red, red lipstick can be a great fashion statement when you're 20. For that matter, so is dramatically bare skin.

As you enter midlife, I want you to set aside your notions of makeup as a camouflage or as a fashion statement and focus on how you can use it to play up your strong points and downplay your weak points.

The biggest mistake that most women make as they age is to wear too much makeup with too little moisturizer underneath. If there's anything worse than parched skin, it's parched skin with caked makeup sitting in the creases.

If you're on a good skin regimen and following the lifestyle changes I've recommended, you should be well on your way to good skin. To play it up with makeup, stick to these strategies.

Less is more. Go heavy on moisturizer and light on base makeup. Use a dampened cosmetic sponge to apply makeup smoothly, and then blend it in with your fingertips. If your skin is really great, skip the base makeup and just use a little concealer where it's needed, diluting it with moisturizer to get a light effect.

Keep your lips natural. Forget about matching your lipstick to the mood of the season or to your outfits— during the daytime, at least. Go for lipstick and lip liner as close as possible to your natural lip color. A little gloss will make your lips look fuller if they're thinning with age. Do not try to alter the shape of your lips with makeup; it looks dated and downright awful. Instead, consider the methods of lip enhancement that I discuss in chapter 10.

Avoid black. Never put anything black on your face if you can avoid it. Even if you used black eyeliner and mascara in your youth, switch to brown in midlife. You'll still get definition without looking like a member of the Addams family as your skin pales with age.

Glow from within. If you must wear blusher, keep it light so you don't end up looking like a painted doll. And never put anything frosted on your eyelids after age 40.

Think of your skin. As with other products, go for cosmetics that are hypoallergenic and noncomedogenic.

Of course, there are exceptions to these principles. But if you follow them, you should be able to achieve a youthful, natural look at any age. Think hard about what you put on your face. I think it was Coco Chanel, the legendary French fashion designer, whose advice regarding jewelry was to put on as much as seems right—and then to take one piece off. If you follow this strategy with your makeup—put on a little less than you think you need—you'll never look overdone.

A Special Look at Acne and Rosacea Therapy: Be Creative

Almost every woman who consults me for acne voices the same frustration: "I'm not a teenager, so why am I still breaking out?"

Contrary to popular belief, acne often persists into adult life and worsens during midlife. That's when some women experience it—or rosacea, acne's cousin—for the first time.

One reason is the hormonal shifts that you may experience from your thirties onward as your body begins to prepare for menopause, 10 to 15 years down the road. In my opinion, the other reason is that midlife is often a period of great physical and psychological stress for women, and one way your skin manifests that stress is as acne.

I'm frequently astounded by the frenetic lives many of my patients lead. More than one has conducted conference calls to the office or discussions with her children's schoolteachers while actually on the exam table, having a procedure done. The most enterprising of all has to be Ariel, a management consultant in her late thirties who successfully (and very vocally) closed a major trans-Atlantic business deal with the aid of the hands-free phone she'd thoughtfully brought along—while I silently gave her a chemical peel.

This may be the time of your life when you're trying to balance the demands of a growing family with the challenges of the wider world. Or when you're finally breaking through the glass ceiling. Or, as it is for many women, the time when it seems you're so busy looking after the health and welfare of everyone around you that you have no time for your own. All this may be unavoidable, but it inevitably takes its toll on your skin.

Adult acne often behaves differently from what we think of as "regular" acne. Instead of the oily skin, blackheads, whiteheads, and pustules that typify teenage acne, you may have red bumps, some of them deep and even painful, around your mouth and on your chin and neck. Your skin may be dry sometimes, rather than oily. Or you may find yourself developing full-blown rosacea, characterized by facial redness, easy flushing, acne bumps, and spider veins.

Acne that's not "typical" may require atypical treatment. If your physician starts you out with the standard acne treatments and you seem to be getting nowhere, then it's time for her to get creative. Your doctor must take your skin type into account when devising a treatment plan for you; otherwise, you could be headed down a frustrating—and potentially disastrous—road.

Azra, a smart and successful cardiologist in her early forties, had consulted another dermatologist about her face before she saw me. He had told her that her acne was "not that bad" and "just a passing phase." She was prescribed an antibiotic solution and Retin-A, which she'd been applying to her skin for a few months when I saw her. It was clear that she was not doing well.

"Nurses and other doctors in the hospital keep asking me why my face is so red," she complained. "It's embarrassing to look like a teenager when I have a floor full of patients to take care of."

Azra had acne, but she also had some of the features of rosacea. Her facial redness had been exacerbated by the drying and irritating effects of the antibiotic and the Retin-A, which were basically acting as Red Flamers. As I've mentioned before, I often see overlap between acne and rosacea in my patients. On top of this, the sparse, deep-seated, and tender acne cysts on her chin had not improved. Adult acne often belies its apparent mildness and requires strong treatment.

The first thing I did was take Azra off everything she was using and put her on Metrolotion, a brand of nondrying antibiotic lotion more commonly used for rosacea than acne. I advised her to use sunscreen every day to avoid flaring of her facial redness. I also recommended Glyderm glycolic acid cleanser for mornings and evenings. (Of course, I chose this cleanser with some caution; you'll recall that glycolic acid can be a Red Flamer. In my experience, this particular cleanser has rarely caused skin irritation, and I felt it was worth a try in Azra because she had the type of acne that might respond well to it.) I also prescribed brand name Bactrim antibiotic pills for her to take twice a day.

Contrary to what you normally hear, acne is the product of inflammation rather than infection. Certain antibiotic pills are effective in treating it because they have strong activity against inflammation. The strategy is to stay on the antibiotics for a few months until the acne has improved as much as possible, then you can come off the pills. I like to do this gradually, rather than stopping the antibiotic suddenly, with the aim of preventing another flare-up.

Happily, Azra was able to tolerate the cleanser, and the effects of this whole regimen were dramatic. Within a couple of months, her facial redness was gone and her skin was clear. After 6 months, she was off the antibiotic pills and still doing well.

Azra had been making 2-hour round trips from her home to my office. I knew how difficult this must be for her with her busy daily schedule, and at this point I suggested that she transfer her care to a local dermatologist. I didn't hear from her for another 8 months and assumed that no news was good news. Then, one day in early spring, she called to tell me that her skin was terrible.

"But what happened?" I asked, surprised. "Things were going fine."

"What happened," Azra replied, "is that the dermatologist you recommended told me that you had put me on the wrong treatment for acne. She insisted that Retin-A was the right treatment and put me back on it. She said I shouldn't be using glycolic acid. What she didn't seem to understand was that it was your 'wrong' treatment that cleared up my skin. And now, after using her 'right' treatment, I'm back to square one. So now I don't care how long it takes me to get to your office. I'm on my way."

The story does have a happy ending; Azra's skin was once again clear within a few months of restarting her previous regimen. And fortunately for her, I opened a new office just a few miles from her home. The moral of this story is not what a wonderful dermatologist I am but that acne at any age, but particularly in midlife, doesn't read the textbooks. If you want your treatment to be successful, look for a doctor with an open mind and the ability to think creatively.

There's another moral, too. I usually discuss follow-up directly with any physician to whom I'm transferring a patient. I didn't do this with Azra. I made the mistaken assumption that Azra, a physician herself, would be an effective advocate for her own medical care. This incident reinforces to me how powerless any woman—even one who's a physician—can feel when placed in the role of a patient.

Never forget or be afraid to be your own advocate for better skin. If what your doctor recommends doesn't make sense or you think she's missing an important point, speak up and say so (politely, of course).

No doctor worth her salt will be offended just because you express your concerns to her. You may be off-track—in which case, she can explain why. But your doctor should be very willing to listen to what you have to say regarding your skin. After all, you've known it longer and better than anyone else.

A Special Look at Excess Hair and Hair Loss: Wanted Dead or Alive

"This is how we know Mother Nature isn't really a woman," I remarked to Felicity. She had just finished telling me about the coarse, dark hairs that were sprouting on her chin. "Or, if she is a woman, she has a strange sense of humor."

If you're losing hair where you want it—on your scalp—and gaining it where you don't—on your face—welcome to the supreme irony of midlife. Again, hormone shifts are responsible. Few women have as full a head of hair at 50 as they did at 25; at the same time, most notice an increase in unwanted hair, particularly on their faces. These changes can be traumatic, as they strike at the very core of a woman's femininity.

If you're experiencing hair loss, a thorough investigation is vital. As you saw from the story of Angela, who overdid the vitamin A, identifying one or two reasons may not be enough. These explanations could simply be masking a more severe underlying problem. I take a detailed medical history, do a full medical examination, and check blood tests on almost every woman who walks into my office with hair loss. If we draw a blank with these investigations, my next step is to perform a scalp biopsy.

I followed this path with Erin. I suspected that her hair shedding was due to her having delivered her son 4 months previously, plus the stress of sleepless nights due to his severe colic. During pregnancy and during times of stress, your hair's normal growth cycle is disrupted. Instead of your having hairs in all stages of the growth cycle, most of them become synchronized in the same stage. This means more hairs than usual eventually enter the shedding stage of their cycle and fall out together, a process known as telogen effluvium.

I administered a tiny shot to numb a small area of Erin's scalp and then painlessly removed a small piece of her scalp skin no bigger than ⅙ inch. When a scalp biopsy is examined under the microscope, it can yield valuable clues about the reason for the hair loss. In Erin's case, the biopsy confirmed my diagnosis, and I was able to reassure her that her hair would eventually regrow, once its growth cycle returned to normal.

If investigations point to a medical cause for the hair loss, removing this cause usually restores hair growth, although it can take 6 to 12 months for you to really notice. I have found Tricomin shampoo and spray, which contain antioxidant copper peptides and special "coating agents" that make your hair fuller, to be useful during this waiting period. In situations where the hair loss truly seems to be a function of age and inheritance, and I can't find any other causes, the shampoo and spray are equally useful. The vast majority of my patients report improvement in their hair, and this treatment has no side effects.

Other remedies for hair loss do exist. For example, stress reduction invariably helps. And over-the-counter **minoxidil** solution (brand name Rogaine) will restore hair in some women. Any hair that regrows will fall out if you stop using the minoxidil, so this is an ongoing, maintenance treatment. Some women who use minoxidil complain of excess facial hair, but this falls out if they stop using the medication. (In chapter 12, I'll discuss a surgical solution for hair loss: hair transplantation.)

A variety of methods can help you deal with unwanted hair. I'll discuss the only two permanent methods—laser hair removal and electrolysis—in chapter 10. Here, I'm going to survey the temporary methods.

Contrary to popular belief, shaving does not make your hair grow back thicker. What it does is make the normally tapered ends of your hairs blunt, so they are more noticeable. Hair-dissolving depilatory creams work well for some women, but they can cause skin irritation.

The Perils of Waxing

If you rely on waxing for hair removal, be aware of what you're letting yourself in for. Waxing rips your hair out of its follicles indiscriminately. When this is done regularly, the repeated trauma can actually distort your hair follicles, giving you ingrown hairs and inflamed red acne-like bumps.

There are two areas of your face that I recommend you never wax. One is your eyebrows, and I'll explain why in chapter 10. The other is your upper lip, where I've noticed that years of waxing can actually cause fine vertical wrinkles similar to the ones that smokers develop.

Does Vaniqa Vanquish Hair?

A new entry in the field of hair removal is the prescription cream Vaniqa, which contains the active ingredient **eflornithine hydrochloride**. It's applied twice a day and blocks hair growth in about half the women who use it. The hair regrows if you stop using the cream. Some of my patients use Vaniqa in conjunction with laser hair removal or other methods. I also find it useful for patients with excess blond or gray hair that does not respond to the hair laser.

Reactions to Skin Care Products

Sometimes it's easy to figure out that you're reacting to a product—you burn or sting soon after you apply it. Sometimes it's not so easy. Marina's face would be fine when she woke up and then get progressively redder as the day wore on. It took her months to realize that she was sensitive to the sunscreen she was religiously applying every morning.

Your skin can take some time to develop an allergy, or you may become allergic to a product when it's reformulated to include new ingredients. That's why the eye cream you used for years without problems may suddenly become the cause of your puffy lids and watering eyes.

Acne and blackheads are perhaps the most insidious of skin reactions because they can occur long after the offending product has become a part of your regular routine. Miriam chalked up her midlife breakouts to hormone fluctuations and stress at work, but her skin cleared when she stopped using the base makeup she'd fallen in love with a couple of years previously.

Samantha's initial sensitivity to a new moisturizer jump-started a much more dramatic—and distressing—condition known as status cosmeticus. Anything she applied to her skin, from cleansers to moisturizer to makeup, caused burning and stinging. "I've tried about 10 brands of soap, and I can't tolerate any of them," she complained. Samantha's skin had launched the ultimate protest, and the only cure was to give it a complete break for several weeks from all skin care products.

Should Your Doctor Sell You Skin Care Products?

The answer to this question is that she should if you think she should, and she shouldn't if you think she shouldn't. It all boils down to common sense.

If your doctor specializes in skin care and performs skin rejuvenation procedures in her office, it makes sense for her to recommend treatments for you to use at home. She will have the requisite knowledge to choose products that will really work for you—hopefully, at a price that works for you too. The results of some procedures, such as chemical peeling or laser resurfacing, can actually be enhanced by using the right at-home regimen before, during, and after the procedure.

I find that dispensing products from my office allows me to control what my patients are using on their skin, which is an essential part of the holistic treatment plans I devise for them. I have far more scientific information about these products than I can get about over-the-counter products. I use and recommend products that I feel will give you better results than you can get over-the-counter.

What doesn't make sense is when a doctor whose specialty has nothing to do with skin dispenses skin products—like Estelle's ophthalmologist. You'd find it pretty peculiar if I suddenly started pushing toothbrushes or eyedrops in my office, so why would you buy a glycolic acid face cream from your dentist or eye doctor?

There's an old joke about dermatology told by specialists in other medical fields. It goes, "If there's something on your skin, rub a bit of steroid in." The joke is meant to imply that there's not a lot to dermatology—just one or two lotions and potions. But the reality is, most other doctors are utterly stumped when it comes to the skin. Many medical students have told me the same thing I had thought to myself as a student: "Skin is the one part of the body we're hardly taught anything about."

A doctor who doesn't specialize in skin is unlikely to be familiar with the research behind issues like the buffering of glycolic acid or the stability of vitamin C, or the latest thinking about antioxidants. And if your doctor doesn't have a complete picture, neither will you. The sad truth is, in these days of falling insurance payments and rising office overheads, many doctors get into the business of marketing skin care products simply to boost their revenues. These medical professionals don't really know any more about what they're hawking than the young woman with bad skin, too much makeup, and a white coat sitting behind a department store cosmetics counter. Sometimes, they know even less.

I urge you to be particularly cautious in situations where an assistant in the doctor's office selects your products without any input from the doctor. Also worthy of suspicion is the doctor's office that carries only multiple products from one brand line, presumably acquired from the first salesman whose company pitch arrived in the right place at the right time. If in doubt, find out. Ask the doctor directly, "What made you start selling skin care products from your office?"

Which Goop Is Worth the Dough?

Forget the adage "You get what you pay for"; when it comes to skin cream, you don't. One of the most expensive over-the-counter youth creams has a lower percentage of active alpha hydroxy acids than its more economical competitors and—at least in my professional experience—is far likelier to cause skin reactions.

What are you really paying for when you buy that $50 cream? Is it the look, the fancy packaging, and the pricey model hired to promote the product in all her airbrushed glory—and the promises that will never come true? If so, you may not hate the model "because she's beautiful"—but you may end up hating her because she just emptied your wallet needlessly.

Some over-the-counter creams really work. Steer clear of the ads for wonder creams that promise to give you baby skin in a matter of days, and instead go for products that contain real therapies, like alpha hydroxy acids or retinol. Instead of being swayed by marketing, look for products backed by solid research that proves they're likely to benefit your skin. Ask the white-coated ladies at the cosmetic counter or in the salon for the concentrations of the active ingredients. If they don't know, they should be able to find out for you. (The concentration of glycolic acid in over-the-counter creams ranges from less than 4 to about 10 percent. But it may be difficult to find out how buffered the cream is—the more buffering, the lower the concentration of active glycolic acid in the cream and the less effective it may be.)

The same issues apply to products you buy in a doctor's office. Often you're paying for a famous name—the one all your friends are talking about because they've been bombarded with the publicity campaign—rather than results. But in the case of these products, details about the active ingredients—for instance, the percentage of glycolic acid or retinoid, or whether the vitamin C is stabilized—should be easier to get. If you don't understand why your doctor is selling you a $100 cream that seems no better than the $40 alternative, don't be afraid to ask why.

Skin on a budget can be every bit as beautiful as its more affluent sisters, if you make the right choices. The over-the-counter picks in my 7-Minute Amazing Skin Regimen cost $5 to $20 each for a month's supply. You may be surprised to learn that skin on a budget can also do very well in a doctor's office. Many of the dispensed products in the 7-Minute Amazing Skin Regimen—and many other products your doctor may dispense—cost about the same as, or little more than, my over-the-counter budget picks. But they have often have higher concentrations of active ingredients, plus sound, proven science to back them up.

My 7-Minute Amazing Skin Regimen

Unless you're a lady who lunches—and late in the day, at that—you may as well forget multistep, elaborate skin routines. The good news is that you can get the same results from a three-step, 7-minute program as you can from one several times longer. All you have to do is to make sure that each step is meaningful.

Of course, there are some optional extras, like toners or masks—if you like them and have the time for them. But when it comes down to it, all skin regimens are basically the same. They clean you, moisturize you, and, hopefully, improve your skin. There's no mystique to the 10-step programs you see at department store cosmetic counters. Often these programs and the puzzling products that comprise them are devised simply to ensure that you buy the maximum number of products.

You really don't need to use separate creams for your throat and your face, or to break open mysterious little capsules to slather their contents under your eyes. All you need is a simple routine that you can follow even when your alarm clock fails to go off and you're running a bit late, when the kids are slower than usual to eat breakfast, or when you get an important phone call just as you've stepped out of the shower. In other words, you need skin care for life—*your* life—every day. I said before, it's consistency that will get you results.

My 7-Minute Amazing Skin Regimen gives you the products that have worked reliably for my patients and are cost-effective. It's no substitute for a dermatological consultation, nor is it a comprehensive guide to every product out there that could help your skin. It's a good starting point if you want to try some over-the-counter products on your own before seeing a doctor—or perhaps you can use it as a guide when your doctor helps you select from products he prescribes or dispenses in his office. And it takes only 7 minutes twice a day.

To use this regimen, first determine whether or not your skin passes the Red Test, which I explained on page 156. If your skin passes, it can probably take alpha hydroxy acids and retinoids without getting irritated or dry, and you can choose either from the products under the heading "If You Pass the Red Test" *or* from the products I've listed as Red Tamers. If your skin flunks the Red Test, choose *only* from the Red Tamers. I've bracketed the active ingredients of each product and listed the skin conditions they can help.

MORNING

Step 1: Cleanser

Never use a washcloth with your cleanser, as harsh rubbing may do much the same as exfoliating scrubs and irritate your skin. It's better to apply your cleanser with gentle, circular motions of your fingers and rinse it off with plenty of comfortably warm or room-temperature water. If you love the quick cleansing and squeaky-clean feeling you get with a washcloth, cleansing cloths are a gentler alternative—although they cost more than a bottle of comparable cleanser. Don't use cleansing pads unless your skin is oily, as they are quite drying.

If You Pass the Red Test

From your doctor:

> *Glyderm, Glytone* or *Topix Glycolix cleanser* or *Topix cleansing pads* (glycolic acid) for wrinkles, discolorations, acne
>
> *Topix Glycolix Gly-Sal pads* (glycolic and salicylic acids) for acne

Over-the-counter:

> *Aqua Glycolic Facial Cleanser* (glycolic acid) for wrinkles, discolorations, acne
>
> *Neutrogena Oil Free Acne Wash* or *Acne Wash Cleansing Cloths* (salicylic acid) for acne

If You Don't Pass the Red Test

From your doctor:

> *Neova Soothing Milk Cleanser* (copper peptide antioxidant) for wrinkles, redness
>
> *Topix Wash Off Cleanser, Topix Non Drying Cleanser* (no active anti-aging or anti-acne ingredients) for general cleansing

Over-the-counter:

> *Cetaphil Gentle Skin Cleanser, Liquid Neutrogena Cleanser, Dove Daily Hydrating Cleansing Cloths* (no active anti-aging or anti-acne ingredients) for general cleansing

Step 2: Cream

Prescription or cosmeceutical creams should generally be applied sparingly. Use the fourth finger of your weaker hand (that's your left hand if you're right-handed) to apply eye cream. Use gentle, circular, patting movements around your eyes, and never pull or drag the delicate skin there. Wait about 2 minutes for creams to be absorbed before proceeding to the next step.

There are several other over-the-counter creams that contain antioxidants. But the active ingredients are frequently mixed with a hodgepodge of other chemicals, making it hard to assess just how much stable, active antioxidant is actually present. The studies that are cited for the effectiveness of these creams tend to focus on visible improvement in skin tone or texture, rather than more objective factors, such as collagen or elastic production. You're probably better off going to your physician for an antioxidant.

If You Pass the Red Test

From your doctor:

Glyderm, Topix Glycolix, or Glytone Facial Creams (glycolic acid) for wrinkles, discolorations, acne; *Glyderm, Topix Glycolix, or Glytone Eye Creams* (glycolic acid) for wrinkles, discolorations, skin firming

Over-the-counter:

Neutrogena Pore Refining Cream (alpha hydroxy acid and retinol) for wrinkles, discolorations, acne, *Neutrogena Healthy Skin Eye Cream* (alpha hydroxy acid and melibiose) for wrinkles, discolorations, skin firming

Aqua Glycolic face cream (glycolic acid) for wrinkles, discolorations, acne

Neutrogena Skin Clearing Moisturizer Daily Face Cream (salicylic acid and retinol) for acne, discolorations

If You Don't Pass the Red Test

From your doctor:

Topix Replenix cream (polyphenol antioxidants) for wrinkles, discolorations, redness; can be used on the face and under eyes

Topix Citrix cream (vitamin C) for wrinkles, discolorations, redness

Neova Eye Therapy (copper peptide antioxidant) for wrinkles, discolorations, skin firming

Glyderm Hydrating Eye Cream (vitamin K) for some improvement of discolorations

Over-the-counter:

> *Neutrogena Healthy Skin Anti-Wrinkle Cream* (retinol) for wrinkles, discolorations, acne
>
> *Almay Kinetin Eye Cream* (furfuryladenine) for discolorations, skin firming
>
> *Neutrogena Visibly Firm Eye Cream* (copper peptide antioxidant) for wrinkles, skin firming

Step 3: Sunscreen

Select a sunscreen that moisturizes your skin adequately, and apply it liberally all over your face and neck, except around your eyes. If you wear makeup, you can apply it about 2 minutes after this step.

From your doctor:

> *Topix Oil-Free SPF 30 Sunblock, Glyderm Super Sunblock SPF 25, ProCyte Ti-Silc SPF 45* (tinted or untinted)

Over-the-counter:

> *Neutrogena Healthy Defense Daily Moisturizer* (SPF 30, tinted or untinted)
>
> *Eucerin Facial Moisturizing Lotion* (SPF 25)

Step 1: Cleanser

Use the same cleanser as you did in the morning.

Step 2: Cream

Use the same eye cream you used in the morning. Use the same face cream you used in the morning, or try one of the following:

If You Pass the Red Test

Prescription:

> *Renova, Avita, or Retin-A cream* (tretinoin) or *Avage cream* (tazarotene) for wrinkles, acne, discolorations, roughness

If You Don't Pass the Red Test

From your doctor or over-the-counter:

Kinerase cream or lotion (furfuryladenine) for wrinkles, discolorations, roughness

Over-the-counter:

Almay Kinetin Night Concentrate (furfuryladenine) for wrinkles, discolorations, roughness

If your skin feels dry after applying Renova, Avita, or Retin-A or Avage, wait a couple of minutes and then apply one of the Red Tamer products to simultaneously moisturize and rejuvenate your skin.

chapter ten

Charms That Heal— Strategies for Successful Cosmetic Procedures

There is no cosmetic for beauty like happiness.

—Marguerite, Countess of Blessington

If there's one thing that predicts whether you'll achieve success from your cosmetic surgery, it's how happy you are going into it. You'd think that any patient who actively seeks and schedules a procedure would, by definition, be happy with what she's doing. But that's not always the case. For instance Sadie, an architect in her mid-forties, insisted that she was "totally ready" for her fat injections but her worried face told me a different story. When I questioned her further, she admitted that she saw her cosmetic surgery as part of her quest to keep up with her sister and that it would squeeze her financially. I immediately advised her not to go ahead with the procedure.

If you want cosmetic surgery to impact your life positively, you must first feel comfortable with your inner Self. What you do on the surface cannot make you feel comfortable with who you are; but it can burnish your inner Self and make it shine brighter. That's what I had to tell Melinda, a 48-year-old interior designer, who called me several times after scheduling her laser resurfacing.

"It makes me feel so old to be doing this," she sighed. "All I need is for you to tell me I'm doing the right thing, and I think I'll be okay."

It never works for a woman to be pushed into cosmetic surgery, even if that push is cloaked in the garb of sympathetic professional advice. In Melinda's case, no number of authoritarian statements from me or any other doctor could solve her fundamental problem: she needed to come to terms with the fact that she was aging. If she didn't, she'd never be able to accept that she would continue to age even after cosmetic surgery. And she'd probably be dissatisfied with her results, no matter how good they were. Laser resurfacing couldn't do anything more than transform her from an unhappy woman with wrinkles into a still-unhappy woman with smoother skin. She needed to achieve inner comfort before embarking on cosmetic surgery.

The key to happiness with cosmetic surgery—as with most things in life—is to figure out your expectations, motivations and anxieties ahead of time. The Red Lights of Beauty in chapter 3 are a good starting point. Then your physician can help you zero in on your most lasting concerns. She should also discuss with you the emotional, physical, and financial aspects of whatever procedures you're considering. That's her responsibility.

But it's *your* responsibility to make sure you get what you want from a consultation. I know this can be difficult if you're conditioned to see your doctor as an authority figure and you feel inhibited even mentioning to her that you just spent 2 long hours in the waiting room. But it's vital that you explore every aspect of the procedures you're contemplating. I urge you not to wall yourself off from the emotional issues, especially if you're considering anything beyond the lightest and most non-invasive cosmetic surgery.

The information that I give you here will help, but you must be your own judge in the end. Your doctor should offer you options but not push you into procedures. If you need more information, don't feel inhibited about saying so. And, above all, don't feel obligated to the doctor you consult. The only obligation you have is to yourself—to make sure that the decision you make is true to your own thoughts, feelings and best judgment. When Denise consulted me, she had recovered recently from a bout of Bell's palsy, a nerve disorder that had suddenly paralyzed one side of her face. Mercifully, the paralysis had vanished after several months, but I could easily appreciate the trauma she'd been through. So it came as no surprise to me when she decided to defer any invasive procedures and stick with facials, eyebrow shaping and an at-home skin care regime for the time being.

"I'm so sorry about this; I've taken up so much of your time discussing all this surgery and now I'm not going to do any of it," she told me sheepishly.

"Denise, there's no need to apologize," I replied. "It's your face and your choice."

As I explained to Denise, any good doctor should accept your decision that a procedure is not for you—and she should understand equally well that talking you into a procedure benefits nobody in the end.

Here, then, are the considerations and strategies you need for successful cosmetic surgery. I'll not only cover the questions you probably have asked already; I'll also deal with some questions that you've not even thought of. That's what I do every day in my practice when I counsel patients regarding their procedural options. And I'll also share with you the stories of women who got what they wanted out of cosmetic procedures—and some who didn't.

Step 1: Know When You're Ready

Linda was concerned that, at 35, she was too young to be thinking about laser resurfacing to improve the lines around her eyes, tighten her jowls, and fade her sunspots. One of the most common questions patients—and potential patients—ask me is "Am I the right age to have cosmetic surgery?"

In fact, there is no "right age." There *is* a right time, but it doesn't depend on your age. The right time to have cosmetic surgery is when something is bothering you, you feel ready to do something about it, and you have realistic goals and expectations. I've fixed the frown lines of 27-year-olds with Botox for whom *this* was the right time. And I've declined to treat 60-year-olds who want the impossible—for laser surgery to make them look 21 again—because this was clearly *not* the right time for them.

Linda got what she wanted from her laser resurfacing because she didn't make the mistake of thinking it would automatically make her a happier—or even more beautiful—person. What she wanted was for her outside appearance to reflect the energy and vigor she felt internally, and she got that. I've treated many patients for whom a life passage—like menopause, the end or beginning of a relationship, turning 40—was the impetus for cosmetic surgery. For Linda, it was the end of her 15-year marriage and the prospect of dating again. Conversely, I've treated as many patients who simply woke up one day and decided they no longer wanted their wrinkles to make them look sad, tired, or angry when they didn't feel that way inside.

And then there are the women who find that cosmetic surgery can actually help them to heal another aspect of their lives.

When Janis came into my office recently, it occurred to me that I hadn't seen this once regular patient in quite a while. One glance at her medical record confirmed that I was correct; her last visit had been more than a year earlier. At that time, she'd been midway through a series of alternating salt macrodermabrasions and glycolic acid chemical peels that was working wonders for her uneven skin tone and adult acne.

"Good to see you," I greeted her. "So we're picking up where we left off?"

"No," replied Janis, her eyes filling with tears. "We're starting over. Since I saw you last, my daughter was killed in a terrible car accident."

You might be shocked to imagine a bereaved mother would have any time or inclination for her appearance. But think back to what I told you about the aftermath of the 9/11 tragedy. In times when we have no control over the larger events in our lives, finding a small aspect that we can control can actually help us to heal.

Of course, I talked to Janis at length to make sure that her decision was rational and that she was emotionally ready to restart her treatment. And as I watched her carefully during her subsequent visits, I was happy to see that her treatment did help her in more ways than by simply clearing her skin. At the very least, she had half an hour's respite every couple of weeks from the memories that pervaded every other corner of her life. And she had the opportunity to think about something unrelated to her tragedy at a time when, as she said, "everyone else I know either turns away from me in embarrassment or can't stop saying how sorry they are."

If you want to know whether *you're* ready, write down your expectations and ask your doctor—and yourself—whether they're realistic. Be honest with yourself about your motivations and anxieties, and be honest with your physician too. Otherwise, you'll waste your time, and you may end up having a procedure that doesn't do you any good.

My acid test for determining whether you're ready is if you feel you *want* cosmetic surgery but don't *need* it. This distinction means you've come to terms emotionally with the fact that cosmetic surgery is always an option but, strictly speaking, one of many. If the only way you can feel comfortable about your decision is to tell yourself it's medically necessary because you're deformed or diseased, well, then, you're not ready.

Step 2: Define Your Problems

One of the biggest mistakes I see women make is getting hung up on specific procedures. They'll ask me, "Is the laser better than a chemical peel?" or "Do you recommend fat injections over Botox?" or "Can you treat me with collagen, because that's what my friend had and she looks great?"

These questions have no general answers. The answers are individual—and conditional—because they depend on what your individual expectations are. For example, if you want to tighten your skin as much as possible and get maximum wrinkle improvement, then yes, laser resurfacing is better for you. Conversely, if you want good results but have to be back at work within 5 days, then you're better off having a chemical peel. If you have a similar pattern of aging and a similar skin type to your friend, then collagen may be the right choice for you too, just as it was for her.

I also caution you against assuming that the procedure you learned about from a magazine or a television program is the one you should have because it's "the newest." Even if a technology is the flavor of this month, that doesn't necessarily mean it's right for you. Your unique pattern of aging doesn't follow trends, nor should you when seeking solutions. In fact, having "the newest treatment" is not always the best option; it could mean you're acting as a guinea pig!

Instead, focus first on your problems. And by "problems," I mean what *you'd* like to fix. Don't let anyone else tell you what to fix—it's only a problem if it bothers *you*. I don't think anyone, even a physician, should define your problems for you. Certainly, take your physician's opinion into account if you've solicited it and you agree with it. But you should always have significant input into the problem-defining process.

I once attended a seminar on nose jobs where the speaker, an ear, nose, and throat specialist, showed a picture of each nose before surgery and labeled it as having a particular "deformity." Most of these noses looked fine to me. They may not have been perfect, but, as I'll tell you on page 188 when I discuss your facial Power Points, there are only three areas of your face where I think it's important to strive for as near perfection as possible. And your nose isn't one of them.

By the end of that seminar, I felt like walking out with my face hidden in my hands. How would a vulnerable patient feel if told authoritatively during a consultation that she had a nose deformity that needed to be cured? I hope she wouldn't rush lemminglike into the nearest operating room or else wallow in deep depression at the thought of her imperfect proboscis.

Once you've defined your problems, then you and your doctor can decide *together* how they will be fixed.

Renata was convinced that she should have laser resurfacing because she'd been told this by other doctors. However, I soon realized that what bothered her most were the deep lines running from the sides of her nose to the corners of her mouth. I've seen innumerable patients with this problem who were bitterly disappointed after the laser resurfacing their doctors prescribed and performed. The best way to fix these lines is with fat injections, which is what I recommended to Renata.

Step 3: Get Over the Guilt

Guilt is an emotion with no positive side. If you want your cosmetic surgery to be successful, you have to stop feeling guilty about it. And to do this, you must understand the reasons for your guilt. I discussed previously why we feel guilty about cosmetic surgery and about beauty itself. Essentially, we're afraid of what others will think if we openly display the desire to look beautiful or to look younger. And we've transferred a lot of the shame it's no longer acceptable to express over sex to the issues of beauty and beauty enhancement.

Rosemary, a retired property developer in her late sixties, is typical of many women I see in my office whose unresolved guilt traps them in the dilemma of indecision. She was delighted with the fat injections I'd used to fill in her smile lines and the chemical peels I'd combined with an at-home regimen of Glyderm glycolic acid cleanser, Claripel hydroquinone cream and sunscreen to lighten her sunspots. She was assiduous about having procedures performed only when her boyfriend was away on business trips because, she said, "He would think I'm so vain if he knew I was doing all this."

All went well for a couple of years. And then, one autumn day, Rosemary's card-house of guilt came tumbling down about her. She was wringing her hands and could hardly suppress her tears as I walked in to see her.

"Doctor, I'm in such big trouble. My boyfriend found your business card; it fell out of my handbag. He told me he'd noticed my freckles were fading and that he hoped I wasn't doing anything to my skin because I would end up deformed. I told him, 'Of course not.' But now I don't know what to do. I'm so pleased with my results and I want to continue. But now I can't. What should I do?"

I told Rosemary that she had two choices. She could give in to her guilt . . . or she could get over it. The one thing she couldn't do was to continue having cosmetic surgery while she felt guilty about it, because she would end up hopelessly conflicted. When Rosemary left my office that day, I didn't know if I'd ever see her again. But she was back a few weeks later, this time with a smile on her face.

Becoming Beautiful without Going Broke

By now, I'm sure you've noticed that many of my patients are pretty down-to-earth. For every so-cialite or millionaire's wife that I treat, there's a teacher, saleswoman, bus driver, or student. That's one of the joys of my profession: bringing the most sophisticated and up-to-date technology to women from every walk of life. I find it both a delight and a challenge to formulate plans of action for these woman and then to see those plans bear fruit in the ensuing weeks, months, or years.

So how do you become beautiful if you haven't broken the bank at Monte Carlo or won the lottery? It's simple. You start with what bothers you the most. If it's your frown lines, fix them first with Botox. This relatively in-expensive treatment yields great re-sults. Then you can move on to your open pores or the drooping at the corners of your mouth. That's what Sandi, my patient who works in a deli, has done. She's become beautiful in stages, and in the process we've gotten to know each other well.

Another strategy is to consider other, less expensive alternatives to your "ideal" procedure. Margot and I both felt that laser resurfacing would be the best way to deal with her wrinkles, loose jowls, and skin discolorations—but in a few years, when her budget allowed it. In the meantime, I started her on antioxidants and glycolic acid at home, and I chemically peeled her face. For a few hundred dollars—one-quarter the cost of laser resur-facing—she had the wrinkle improvement and skin tightening she needed to see her through until she was ready for her definitive procedure.

Ana was dismayed at the cost of blepharoplasty—surgical tight-ening of her eyelids. But she left my office smiling after eyebrow reshaping, which didn't cure her drooping eyelids but made them much less noticeable and drew at-tention instead to her lustrous, al-mond-shaped eyes. The cost? Twenty dollars, as opposed to the thousands she'd have spent on a blepharoplasty.

"I talked it over with my boyfriend," she told me. "I just took a deep breath and told him what I was doing. And, you know what, he wasn't shocked. He just didn't want me to be doing things without telling him. But he also doesn't want to see me peeling or with marks on my face," she continued with a laugh, "so let's keep doing it while he's out of town!"

Guilt is not always as easily resolved as it was for Rosemary. Sometimes it's so deeply embedded in your psyche that you have to scrutinize yourself very carefully to understand it. I think it helps to write down your concerns. When you put your guilt into words, it is demystified and you are forced to confront it in concrete form, rather than as a nebulous concept. Remember Nia? She's my patient who'd developed a double chin during her pregnancy and who felt guilty about seeking liposuction because it was "unnatural." Nia got over her guilt by realizing that it was irrational, because she'd already enhanced her beauty by other "unnatural" means like orthodontic teeth-straightening and eyebrow-shaping. The simple act of listing these other beauty-enhancing procedures and describing their positive effects helped her to make a rational, fact-based decision about her liposuction.

Step 4: Play to Your Strengths

Unless you're fabulously wealthy and have large amounts of free time on your hands, chances are you're going to have to be selective about what you want to do with your face. Or, at the very least, you need to decide on a starting point. My advice to you is play to your strengths. Figure out, with the help of your doctor, which are your face's high points, and then make a plan to balance the rest of your face so these high points can shine.

Let me give you an example. Rachel is not classically beautiful, but she has strikingly large, deep blue eyes. When she asked which one procedure would make the most difference to her appearance, I didn't hesitate to recommend that she have her lips enhanced. They'd always been thin but had become more so as she had entered her mid-forties.

"The fat injections in your lips will be subtle, and people won't even guess you've had something done," I predicted. "But what they will notice more is your eyes because your whole face will be rebalanced."

Sure enough, Rachel has even been stopped by strangers on the street since her fat injections, and they all sing the praises of "those gorgeous eyes."

To understand how playing to your strengths works, look at another woman's face and notice how your gaze is drawn to the weak points; the crow's-feet around her eyes, the puckering of her lips, or her frown lines. These weak points often distract you from seeing the good points. That's what was happening to Rachel; nobody appreciated her spectacular eyes because they were focusing on her aging mouth. Once I fixed her lips, everyone's gaze was directed upward, to her eyes.

Every face has strengths. The trick is to find them and to understand how to play them up. To do this, you often need to improve one or more of your three power points to balance your face.

Step 5: Know Your Power Points

Giving careful attention to the three power points is one of the most important principles I use in my cosmetic surgery. As we've discussed, a face that's totally symmetrical is often not as appealing as one with slight asymmetries. A little imperfection is beautiful because it makes you human, whereas a totally symmetrical face tends to look impersonal and devoid of emotion. But there are three areas of your face where it's worthwhile for you and your doctor to aim for as close to perfection as you can. Making these power points as symmetrical as possible will optimize your beauty without stripping it of its individuality.

The important thing to realize about your power points is that all can be improved relatively easily. You don't have to be born with great skin or great eyebrows—they can be acquired. Some of us are naturally blessed with better lips than others. But these days, thanks to injections of collagen or fat, turning ordinary lips into extraordinary ones—if that's what you yearn for—is simply a matter of minutes.

Power Point 1: Your Skin

Think of your skin as the canvas of your face and the foundation of your beauty. To appreciate how important your skin is to your looks, think of what would happen if you tried to paint a portrait on a substandard canvas. No matter how good the quality of your brushwork, the painting would suffer. That's what happened to the Renaissance painter and philosopher Leonardo da Vinci, who placed an exquisite painting, *The Last Supper*, directly onto the wrong base: dry plaster. The shortcomings of this plaster base doomed the oil painting to perpetual imperfection, necessitating restoration work even during his lifetime and several times since then.

When I first saw Monica, the manager of a prominent local beauty salon, I could immediately see that she was doing a da Vinci. Her painstakingly made-up face and immaculately coiffed hair couldn't hide the fact that her skin was in distress. I felt pretty certain that her complaint of puffy red eyelids was not her only problem and that she had serious skin redness and flaking lurking beneath the layers of makeup on her cheeks and chin. But when I asked Monica to wash her face so that I could examine it, she froze in her chair.

"I only want you to look at my eyelids," she retorted. "My skin's fine; I use all-natural European products and makeup from my salon."

I looked at her but said nothing. As a partly European-trained physician myself, I could have told Monica that face creams that have crossed the Atlantic boast nothing intrinsically superior—they're just as likely to cause a skin reaction as their American cousins. Some natural products *cause* skin rashes. A number of botanical extracts contain chemicals that irritate your skin, make it sensitive to the sun, or cause skin allergies. Still, Monica's defensive posture—her arms crossed tightly across her chest and her shoulders hunched over her knees—made it clear that she was in no mood to listen to all this.

I sent her away with a mild prescription cortisone cream as a temporary fix for her eyelid rash and asked her to return for allergy testing. I had a strong suspicion that her problem was due to a reaction to one of her facial products or even to her nail polish. Allergy to nail polish often shows up on our eyelids. We all unconsciously touch our faces with our fingers innumerable times during the day, and the thin, delicate skin of our eyelids is more likely show an allergic reaction then the more robust parts of our faces.

The allergy testing, known as patch testing, was painless. I applied two self-adhesive paper strips to Monica's back. These strips were impregnated with the 24 substances that account for the vast majority of skin allergies. Monica kept her back dry for 2 days and then returned to my office so I could read the patch test.

The test showed that Monica was highly allergic to fragrances and to nickel, a white metal found in some jewelry and watch straps and in some metal objects (like eyebrow tweezers) that may touch your face. "Your allergies may well be the cause of your rash," I explained to Monica. "The only way to find out if they are is to avoid what you're allergic to. That means no products containing perfume."

Monica shook her head decisively at this. "You don't understand. All the products in my salon contain an exclusive French perfume. I have to set an example by wearing my own products so that my clients will buy them."

I resisted the temptation to point out that anyone looking at Monica's skin would hardly be persuaded to use what she was using. Instead, I decided to set the fragrance issue aside temporarily and move on to the nickel. Monica already knew she reacted to costume jewelry. She avoided it assiduously and wore only gold ornaments. But I thought the source of her eyelid rash lay literally in her hands. Monica used an eyelash curler every morning. And metallic beauty gadgets like curlers, tweezers, and bobby pins often contain nickel.

I'd like to say that Monica eventually saw the light, removed fragrance and nickel from her life, and cleared her skin. But, sadly, that's not the case. On subsequent visits to my office, she steadfastly refused even to let me see her face without makeup and insisted that she had to keep using the same products for the sake of her business. I think she felt uneasy about exposing her vulnerabilities as a skin care expert to me. The last time I saw her, her makeup was thicker than ever, and her skin was still protesting.

Flawless skin does not exist outside of an airbrushed magazine cover. But you actually don't even need to come close to flawless. Good skin that glows with health is so rare at any age that, should you achieve it, you'll stand out in every crowd. The point of healthy skin is that it's more than a canvas for makeup. Healthy skin is the work of art itself and the other facets of your beauty are accents for it.

If you follow the guidelines in this book, work from the inside out, establish a simple but regular at-home skin regimen and seek professional help when you want it, it's well within your grasp to have the perfect canvas for your beauty.

Power Point 2: Your Eyebrows

"You've got to help me!" Paulette exclaimed, despair clouding her normally happy features. I was instantly transported back to 4 years earlier, when Paulette, an events planner in her thirties, had told me exactly the same thing. Back then, a little Botox had smoothed her brow and allowed her to sail self-confidently through her first dinner with her boyfriend's parents. Now she and that boyfriend were newlyweds and due to attend a family reunion.

The problem was an eyebrow shaping she'd received at a well-known local salon by a beautician a local magazine had recommended as "the best in town." He had waxed and tweezed Paulette's eyebrows and then trimmed them with scissors. The results were disastrous. She had the typical results of waxing: her brows were too flat in the middle, too thin at the sides, and ended too abruptly at both ends. She also had a tell-tale zone of lighter-colored skin just above her brows, where the wax had been applied and stripped off. To make matters worse, her eyebrows had somehow been tweezed and trimmed into points, giving her face a disturbingly pixielike look. And her left eyebrow was distinctly fuller in the center than her right.

"I going to be meeting John's aunt and several of his cousins for the first time—and look at me!" she lamented.

I shook my head in sympathy; I wasn't sure that even Mirvia, my eyebrow shaping specialist, could do anything much until Paulette's eyebrows had grown out for a week or two.

"But we're flying to Florida tomorrow! Can't she at least try?" Paulette pleaded.

Luckily, the story has a happy ending. As so often, Mirvia amazed me—and my patient. She smoothed out the pixie points, evened the asymmetry, and restored at least some of the arch to Paulette's brows so that she could attend the family reunion without embarrassment. And when she returned to my office a few weeks later, her brows had grown out enough for perfect shaping.

If your eyes are the window to your soul, your eyebrows are surely their frame. The first thing to understand is that it's virtually impossible for you to perfect that frame yourself. The reason for this is simple: You cannot see your face in three dimensions. Brows that look great to you when you see yourself front-on can look downright terrible from the side. Good eyebrows can truly make your face—and bad ones can break them.

What are good eyebrows? To paraphrase a famous legal judgment about pornography, they're difficult to describe, but I know them when I see them. Good eyebrows curve gracefully across your face, subtly tapering from middle to ends. They are at once feathery and well-defined. And above all, they soulfully enhance and draw attention to your eyes.

I'm convinced that eyebrow shaping is a gift you have to be born with. It's not just a matter of having good manual dexterity and a steady hand. A truly gifted eyebrow shaper also needs an infallible eye and artistic vision. I liken the talent to a sculptor's ability to see the beautiful finished form that lies within a rough-hewn block of marble.

Only three methods exist that can give you perfect brows—and, of these, only two that I wholeheartedly recommend. The first method is to tweeze the hairs individually under the guidance of a magnifying lens, and that's what Mirvia does. This takes immense skill, but it's painless, and the results are stunning if you can find someone who's really good.

The second method is threading, which I highly recommend to you as a great spectator sport if you're ever in the Far or Middle East. It's amazing to see the precision with which a skilled practitioner of this ancient art can wrap a cotton thread around single hairs and whisk them out swiftly and almost painlessly.

I vividly remember having my eyebrows threaded for the first time in India several years ago. The light was dim, and the entire procedure—performed by a woman who scarcely seemed to glance at me as she was working—took no more than 1 minute. I was so sure that the results would be disastrous that I ran straight back to the house where I was staying. Only then did I dare to look in the mirror, and I discovered that my brows were breathtakingly perfect. Unfortunately, finding anyone in this country who threads well is difficult, if not impossible. Eyebrows threaded here tend to end up too flat in the middle and too thin at the ends—basically the same problems that occur with waxing.

The third method is electrolysis, in which a needle is passed down the side of each hair to reach its root, which lies inside the tubelike hair follicle. An electric current is applied to the hair root to destroy it. This lengthy process can take several sessions over a few months. Electrolysis is permanent, so before embarking on the initial treatment, make absolutely sure that it will be performed by the right person. Keep in mind also the risk inherent to having your brows shaped by electrolysis: brows that are perfect for you at 30 will probably *not* be perfect as your face ages. In general, you need to arch your eyebrows a little higher as you get older, to offset their tendency to flatten and fall with age. (More on this in chapter 12.) You can't have them reshaped to counterbalance these changes if they've already been shaped permanently. This immutability is the biggest reason I have reservations about recommending electrolysis for your eyebrows.

Most salons wax brows, for one simple reason: low cost. Waxing takes only a few minutes, so it's very cost-effective. You will never achieve perfect brows by waxing, however, because it's too imprecise a method. Beware of anyone who tells you—as a beautician told one of my patients recently after waxing her—that eyebrows are "supposed" to be uneven. And don't let anyone ever trim your brows with scissors because they're "too long." Length gives your brows their natural beauty.

I urge you to see for yourself how skilled eyebrow shaping—which generally costs no more than $20 or $30—can transform your face. Unfortunately, you may have to resort to some trial and error before you find a good eyebrow shaper; she could be anywhere from your local salon to your doctor's office. But try to get a word-of-mouth recommendation if you can, and make sure you see the brows of the person whose word you're taking. And if you meet anyone with eyebrows to die for, don't feel shy about asking where she got them!

Power Point 3: Your Lips

The ideal lips of today are not the ideal lips of yesteryear. Over the past 3 decades, we've steadily favored fuller and fuller lips. This change may be a reflection of increasing ethnic diversity. The preference for fuller lips is also evolutionarily sound. Full lips are reminiscent of sexual arousal and thus fulfill one of our most important criteria for beauty.

Some of my Black or Latin patients find it amusing that they're now feted for what they were previously faulted. As Amy, who's African-American, mused: "What goes 'round comes 'round! *Everyone* admires my mouth these days."

If your skin is the canvas for your beauty and your eyebrows are the frame, then your lips are the centerpiece. Watch yourself and others, and see how our eyes are inexorably drawn to the mouths of those we meet. Perfect lips can be hypnotically beautiful. They compensate for any number of imperfections on your face. And, like any centerpiece, they highlight the beauty of what's around them.

Think of blue-eyed Rachel. After the fat injections into her lips, one of her friends even asked her if she'd started wearing colored contact lenses; evidently, he'd never really noticed her eyes until her lips were enhanced!

Lip enhancement is also fun and often lifts patients' spirits like no other procedure. I'll always remember Moira, an accountant in her mid-forties, whose entire personality seemed to change after I injected her lips with collagen. She was transformed from the epitome of staidness into a master of zingy one-liners. And her wardrobe reflected this change too, as she swapped her tasteful but conservative strands of pearls for adventurous pendants gleaned from craft shows.

By lip enhancement, I don't mean what you may be thinking. Strike from your mind the image of Goldie Hawn's pneumatically inflated mouth in *First Wives Club*. Or the vision of countless Hollywood starlets with over-the-top (and outrageously over-the-teeth) mouths that seem to have a life of their own. I think the best lip enhancement is subtle and undetectable. To my knowledge, not one of my patients has ever had a finger pointed at them and been told, "You've had your lips done!" The closest anyone's come is to compliment them on their lipstick ("Have you changed your shade?") or, quite simply, to sigh, "You have the most gorgeous lips!"

Some women come to me seeking changes that I know will not benefit them. Often what they want to improve will not impact their facial power points. For instance, Giulia, a student nurse, hated her rounded face because it made her look like a teenager instead of a woman in her mid-twenties. She was convinced that liposuction of her cheeks would solve the problem, but I felt otherwise.

"You're going to be so glad of those cheeks when you're 40," I explained. "Everyone's face gets thinner with time—especially if they have high cheekbones, as you do. Your cheeks will keep you looking young. Liposuction would be the biggest mistake you could make."

"But I've read about movie stars having cheek liposuction," Giulia protested.

"Yes, that was the vogue several years ago," I replied. "And now the people who had it done look like corpses and are having fat injections to restore what they had taken away. If you want to draw attention away from your cheeks, I'd suggest *adding* fat—or collagen—to your lips."

Giulia's lips had a good Cupid's bow, but her upper lip was much thinner than her lower lip. Correcting this power point asymmetry with collagen injections brought out the full beauty of her lips and, as I had promised her, streamlined her whole face. Giulia still looked young for her age, but she now had a new air of sophistication. "It's great!" she told me with a smile. "My baby face just grew up a little."

Over the years, I've found that the power point approach works consistently well. I find it a surefire method for achieving natural-looking beauty from cosmetic surgery and avoiding the overdone, Barbie doll look.

Step 6: Have the Serenity to Accept What You Can't Change and the Courage to Change What You Can

. . . And the wisdom to know the difference. The advice of the old serenity prayer is timeless—and priceless. Certain things about your appearance at any age simply must be accepted because they cannot be changed. Or, more to the point, you need to accept these aspects of your appearance because they cannot be changed *well* and because changing them might rob you of the individuality that makes every face unique.

If you don't like your nose or your cheeks or your chin, there's no limit to what you can do to them these days. But proceed with caution, or you may get more than you bargained for. Think of Coco Chanel and do just a little less than you feel is necessary.

Daria was the epitome of Persian beauty, with her luxuriant, chiseled eyebrows and smooth golden complexion. She was pleased with the laser treatments I'd performed to rid her of the unwanted hair, on her upper lip and cheeks, that had embarrassed her since childhood. But she was unhappy with her dramatic profile, particularly the curve of her nose, which she complained made her look like a hawk. She talked to several plastic surgeons about a rhinoplasty—a nose job—and finally settled on one whom she felt understood what she wanted.

But her new nose was a bitter disappointment. Slightly upturned and blunt-tipped, it might have been great for a delicate-featured blonde—although, even there, it would have been a little too pert for my liking. But it was a disaster, stuck in the middle of Daria's exotic features, where it reminded me of a daisy in a field of orchids.

Like Daria, many of us are societally conditioned to strive for what we think is "normal." But there is no "normal" beauty in real life. You'll probably be viewed as beautiful if you possess certain facial features and your power points are strong. But that still gives your face plenty of latitude for variation in other departments. If someone described you as looking "extraordinary," you'd be happy, right? Well, extraordinary literally means that you are "out of the ordinary," or *not* normal.

When you're considering a cosmetic procedure, lose your fear of not being "normal," keep in mind what makes *your* face extraordinary, and have the courage to avoid changing it. Otherwise, you may wake up from your procedure and find you've been molded into the plasticized perfection that passes for beauty in some social and geographical circles.

Sometimes changing takes as much courage as resisting change. Ellen was making plans for her fourth and final turn as the mother of the bride. Her husband and three older daughters told her she looked wonderful as she was. Her youngest daughter, the bride-to-be, begged her not to change anything—because "I don't want you to look different."

But Ellen had another image in her mind. An avid tennis player and mall walker even at 70, she'd already picked out the dress she would wear to the wedding. Her simple but elegant fitted gown boasted beige lace with a scooped neck that charmingly displayed her petite physique. And she had one accessory she didn't want: years' worth of sun damage on her face, neck, and chest.

I was able to reverse much of this sun damage with laser resurfacing. Her wrinkles and sunspots faded dramatically, and her skin was noticeably tighter. But of course she still looked like the mature woman she was, which was fine with her. I had discussed her likely results with her at length before the procedure and made sure she knew what to expect.

Ellen was the ideal candidate for cosmetic surgery because she was comfortable with her age *and* with her wrinkles. She simply wanted to turn back the clock a little. She was delighted with the results, even more so when her local sandwich shop refused to give her a seniors' discount because she didn't look old enough.

"Now, this is one side effect I *love!*" she told me with a grin.

Ellen's family was thrilled too. As her youngest daughter put it, "You still look like Mom—only better." And her husband, a retired engineer who'd been keenly interested in the laser physics used to rejuvenate his wife, was so impressed that he presented me with copies of the before and after photos he'd taken himself.

From time to time, I pull out those photos, and I'm astounded at just how much improvement Ellen achieved. The rejuvenation of her skin is dramatic, and at first glance even her eyes seem to have changed—they look so much more peaceful. A closer look reveals why. Before surgery, the serenity in Ellen's pastel blue eyes seemed out of place in its weather-beaten surroundings. But afterward, her eyes are perfectly in harmony with the softened contours of her revitalized face. The effect is stunning.

chapter eleven

Caveat Emptor! Strategies for Choosing a Cosmetic Surgeon

The only tyrant I accept in this world is the still voice within.

—Mahatma Gandhi

urn on the radio, open a magazine, or sort through your mail, and you'll probably be bombarded with advertisements for cosmetic surgeons and the procedures they perform. Having so much choice is great, but it can also be quite bewildering. Most of the advertisements make the same offers—the best doctor, the best equipment, and the best result possible. You also might have the doctor who's been referred by word of mouth, by your friend, an acquaintance, or another physician.

Make no mistake; finding the doctor who's right for you is one of the most important parts of the whole cosmetic surgery equation, and also one of the most frightening. I've read several horror stories about patients whose cosmetic surgery went disastrously wrong, causing them humiliation, injury, or even death. When you read these stories as a po-

Caveat Emptor! Strategies for Choosing a Cosmetic Surgeon

199

tential patient, it may seem to you that cosmetic surgery is an unpredictable, high-stakes gamble.

As a physician, I have quite a different perspective when I read those stories. Cosmetic surgery has established safety and competence guidelines, just as there are guidelines for removing your appendix or your ingrown toenail. When these guidelines are flouted or ignored, problems arise. All the horror stories I've read had one basic root cause: the wrong surgeon.

In the previous chapter, I discussed the mindset I believe is most likely to make your cosmetic surgery successful. In this chapter, I'm going to move on to the next step and guide you in selecting the right surgeon. I've summarized below what I feel you need to know to choose the woman or man who will translate your dreams into reality. I hope this information will relieve the feeling that you're working in the dark and put you in control of that all-important selection process. First, though, I'd like you to read a story that spells out exactly why selecting the right physician is such a critical step. Don't let this happen to you!

A Cautionary Tale of Lindsay and the Laser

Lindsay was a beautician who, at age 27, had already had breast implants and extensive liposuction. We met a week after a surgeon had treated two chickenpox scars on her left cheek with laser resurfacing because Lindsay was concerned that her skin was not healing well.

"My doctor told me it was a bacterial infection, and he gave me these antibiotics," Lindsay said, pulling a bottle from her handbag. "But all they did was give me a yeast infection, and my skin's no better."

The treated area on Lindsay's cheek was yellow and crusted. I could easily see how a doctor who was unfamiliar with the skin might mistakenly think this was impetigo, a highly contagious bacterial infection. But closer inspection led me to a different conclusion. There were one or two tiny fluid-filled blisters within the crusted area, and I immediately suspected that this was a viral infection, which would not respond to antibiotics.

You may be surprised to know that you can unknowingly harbor the cold sore virus, even though you may never have experienced a cold sore. It's so easy to pick up this virus in childhood or young adulthood. The virus then hibernates within the roots of the nerves that connect to your skin, and it can awaken from hibernation—a process known as re-activation—and cause cold sores if your skin is injured or if you're sick, under stress, menstruating, or exposed to strong sunlight.

In Lindsay's case, I suspected that the laser treatment had reactivated the virus. This occurs commonly enough that I—and any other experi-enced cosmetic surgeon—routinely give patients medication to prevent virus reactivation when they're having laser resurfacing or chemical peels. I start this treatment a couple of days before the procedure and continue it until the skin is completely healed.

"But my doctor never did that!" Lindsay replied when I explained all this to her.

Looking at Lindsay's cheek, I could see we had no time to lose. She was at great risk of developing disfiguring scars unless I acted quickly. I swabbed her cheek for a viral culture but started her immediately on an-tiviral medication, knowing that it could be too late if I waited for the cul-ture result.

Happily, Lindsay's skin cleared completely and dramatically. And the culture was positive for the cold sore virus I had suspected. Lindsay was delighted and relieved, but she was not so thrilled with her laser surgery.

"The scars are still there. I can't stand them; they make me look hideous. Can you please laser me again?" she pleaded.

I examined her face. Even I, with sharp eyesight, could barely see the scars on Lindsay's stunningly attractive face. Each was no larger than a grain of salt. Lindsay's self-image and expectations were patently unre-alistic. I would never have agreed to treat her the first time, and I certainly wasn't about to treat her the second time around.

Lindsay was bitterly disappointed when I told her this, and she firmly rejected my suggestion to seek counseling regarding her self-image. Unfortunately, she soon found another surgeon to laser her face again. This time she did take antiviral medication, but she was equally unhappy with the laser treatment.

As she stood in my office, complaining about her latest experience, I was hit by a sudden thought. The best way to judge a cosmetic surgeon may be to simply ask, "Do you treat every patient who wants to be

Caveat Emptor! Strategies for Choosing a Cosmetic Surgeon

201

treated?" Because at the end of the day, it's the patients a doctor *doesn't* treat—and the reasons she chooses not to treat them—that really show she knows what she's doing.

Enough of the scary stuff. You know now what can go wrong, so let's focus on how to find the *right* doctor for you.

The ABCs of Finding the Right Doctor for You: Ability, Board Certification and Chemistry

Let's assume some basics: your doctor's office is clean, his general demeanor meets with your approval, and his staff is courteous. Done? Okay, then you're ready to move on.

The first area to focus on is his **ability**. Ask him how much experience he's had with the procedures you're discussing and what his results have been. Many doctors like to show you "before" and "after" pictures of other patients, with the aim of displaying their ability. These photos are useful, up to a point. Seeing how somebody with similar concerns fared can be informative and fascinating. But bear in mind that a doctor will show you his *best* results—it's only human nature. His triumphant photos may not be typical of all his patients.

Before and after pictures carry a new caveat these days. Many companies that sell lasers and other equipment to doctors also provide them with albums containing before and after shots. So it's worth asking your doctor if he himself achieved the impressive results he's showing you, or if the photos are part of a company's publicity kit.

How about computer imaging? Two types exist. The first is simply a digitalized on-screen version of before and after photos. This is slicker and sexier, but basically the same as, the doctor's handing you a few Polaroids.

The second type of computer imaging attempts to show you how you would look if you had a particular procedure. You can see two images alongside each other on the monitor screen: yourself as you are and yourself as you could be. Note that I say "could be" and not "will be." The after image is your doctor's best guess at how his surgery will turn out. How good a guesser he is depends on his ability and experience. Notice how you can find yourself in a circular situation? To judge your doctor's ability, you're evaluating images whose reliability depends upon your doctor's ability.

That's why I'm not a particular fan of computer imaging. These photos can be misleading to patients because they put the veneer of objectivity ("This is how you'll look") on a process that is in reality profoundly subjective ("This is how I think you'll look"). If I feed your picture into a laser surgery imaging program, I can set it to show you with 50 percent, 70 percent, or even 90 percent improvement after the procedure I propose to perform. Despite the handy percentages, there's nothing scientific about this; I'm selecting a figure based solely on my whim.

Another reason that computer imaging may be less than helpful is that it allows your doctor to sidestep the process of communicating with you. For many doctors, actually speaking with their patients is the hardest part of the consultation because it requires social skills and time. And, as you'll know if you've visited doctors recently, it can be tough to find one with either, let alone both.

I recently called for the first time on an ear, nose, and throat physician who was the friend of a friend. He shook my hand and led me into his office, where he asked me a few questions about myself and my training, while barely maintaining any eye contact. Then, without further ado, he sat down, turned on his computer, and began to show me his before and after shots while his nurse leaned over his shoulder and piped in with her remarks during his running commentary. Don't get me wrong; the pictures were quite impressive, and I'd certainly consider referring patients to him for nose jobs. But what struck me was that this must be his *modus operandi* with patients.

From your point of view, it's vital that your doctor actually talk to you face-to-face, rather than fob you off onto an assistant or blind you with technology. In the end, when you're in the procedure room, the relationship that really matters is the one you have with your doctor, not with his nurse or with his computer.

In my opinion, you can best assess a doctor's ability the good, old-fashioned way: by asking to speak to patients who've already gone through the procedure. This gives you so much more information than a mute, two-dimensional image. Your doctor should be able to arrange for one or more of his previous patients to call you—that way, they can stay

Caveat Emptor! Strategies for Choosing a Cosmetic Surgeon

203

anonymous if they wish. What questions should you ask a patient who calls you? Anything you'd like to know, beginning with:

◆ Were you happy with the doctor?
◆ Were you happy with his staff?
◆ Were you happy with your results?
◆ Were there any complications?
◆ What was the best part of the procedure?
◆ What was the worst part of the procedure?
◆ Knowing what you know now, would you have the procedure again with this doctor?

The B of the ABCs is **board certification**. A physician who is board-certified in a particular medical specialty has completed the required years of training and then passed an exam intended to test her knowledge of that specialty. There's much more to being a good doctor than just board certification. Nonetheless, it's a pretty good yardstick to ascertain that your doctor is trained to a generally accepted level. These days, the fastest and most reliable way to verify a doctor's board certification is go on-line to the web site of the medical board in the state where your doctor practices. This web site will also give you information about his training and qualifications, and whether the medical board has ever taken disciplinary action against him.

If you've made sure your doctor is board-certified, the next question is, in what field? Like many patients, you may be surprised to discover that any physician can set up shop as a cosmetic surgeon tomorrow if she desires, regardless of the field in which she was trained. And many do. You don't have to be a dermatologist to be a skin rejuvenation expert—many plastic surgeons and some physicians of other specialties have the requisite experience—but it helps. The challenge for you is to make sure that your physician is properly qualified to perform the procedures she's discussing.

Several years ago, I was teaching a course in laser resurfacing to a group of doctors who were interested in purchasing laser equipment. I explained the physics of the laser and then began to discuss the method of treatment. I mentioned that it was essential to remove skin cells all the way down to the dermis, which, as you'll recall, is the second layer of your skin. At this, one of the attendees—a board-certified family practitioner—raised his hand and asked me, "What's the dermis?"

Why would a family practitioner with no knowledge of even the most basic skin anatomy want to laser your face? He was actually planning to perform laser surgery in the same room where he took Pap smears—a nightmare scenario in terms of infection risk!

One more word about board certification: Many plastic surgeons state in their advertisements that only a board-certified plastic surgeon should be performing a particular procedure. Often this statement is in reference to liposuction. This is ironic, given the fact that the current method of liposuction used by physicians of all specialties, including plastic surgery, was actually developed and refined by a dermatologist, not a plastic surgeon. When physicians of a certain specialty try to claim a procedure as exclusively theirs and represent physicians of other specialties as invaders or intruders, you're witnessing a turf battle that can only confuse and frighten patients needlessly. Don't let turf battles muddy the waters for you when you're selecting a surgeon. (For an explanation of the difference between a plastic surgeon and a cosmetic dermatologist, see the box on page 212, "Know Your Docs.")

If your doctor tells you she's board-certified, ask, "In what field?" Integrate this knowledge with the information you've gathered about your doctor's experience, and use your common sense. If it doesn't seem right to you that your doctor should be doing a particular procedure, then it isn't right. You wouldn't want a board-certified dermatologist, like me, to deliver babies (it's been 14 years since I last had that pleasure). So why would you let a board-certified OB/GYN inject your leg veins—as happens at some vein clinics—or let a family practitioner laser your face?

The final element of the ABCs is **chemistry**. Your doctor may be supremely qualified and competent, but does he *feel* right to you? You must go with your gut instincts in this respect. Cosmetic surgery is an enormous emotional investment, and you've got to feel comfortable turning to your doctor at any time if you have questions or concerns. This familiarity and comfort can develop only when you have a good rapport.

One common mistake is for patients to assume that a doctor's bedside manner doesn't matter if he's a good surgeon. Maybe this is okay 95 percent of the time, when everything goes smoothly (although I'd argue that

Caveat Emptor! Strategies for Choosing a Cosmetic Surgeon

205

you're still better off with a doctor you can relate to). But if you have a complication from your procedure, your lack of chemistry with your doctor can be a major disaster. If your doctor doesn't seem interested in listening to you before surgery, assume that this will also be the case afterwards.

I know because I speak from personal experience. A few years ago, I consulted a well-known ophthalmologist about LASIK laser vision correction. As a rule, patients did not meet him before surgery; they were seen and evaluated by his staff and would meet the doctor for the first time a couple of minutes before the actual procedure. However, at my special request, I did get to meet the doctor about a month before my surgery.

I'm sure he was a great surgeon, but his bedside manner was nonexistent. He spent the entire 6-minute consultation backing away from me with his hand on the door handle. I'd done a fair amount of reading and research myself about the LASIK procedure, so I had only a couple of questions. But he did not seem at all interested in answering them.

The surgery was uneventful. But when I developed a complication afterward, the doctor was nowhere to be found. His staff told me that he was "too busy"! And his partner ended up treating me for the complication until it resolved. The doctor who had performed my procedure—and charged me several thousand dollars for it—couldn't even pick up the phone and talk to me for a couple of minutes when I needed his input.

I hear stories like this every week from patients in my office. The bottom line is, surgical expertise and bedside manner are *not* mutually exclusive. And don't just stop with simple bedside manner. Your doctor's communication skills may be irreproachable, but you and he may simply not be on the same wavelength. If you don't find what you want in the first, second, or even the third doctor you meet, keep looking.

Some cosmetic surgeons charge a fee for an initial consultation—generally in the range of $50 to $150—and some don't. But don't talk yourself into choosing a doctor to perform your procedure just because you paid to consult with him. This would be penny-wise and pound-foolish. If a cosmetic surgery consultation leaves you cold for any reason, the fee you paid to discover this is money well spent.

I've urged you to avoid overfocusing on perfection from your cosmetic surgery itself. But you're entitled to as close to perfect a match as possible when it comes to your physician. Don't turn yourself into a victim for fear of what a doctor will think if you don't choose him for your procedure. You have the right to ask questions and to demand the best. And you—not your best friend or your neighbor or that magazine you skimmed in the supermarket checkout line—are the sole arbiter of what's best for you.

Is Your Doctor's Heart in It?

Beyond looking at the ABCs, one of the most important questions you can ask your doctor is "Why did you choose this field?" Ask this question of a physician who chose cosmetic surgery for the right reasons, and you will see the answer in her eyes—because it's what she loves to do.

One of the most disturbing trends in cosmetic surgery is the tendency to regard it as some sort of medical gold mine or business strategy in an era of falling insurance payments. In doing so, doctors lose sight of the fact that we are not dealing in commodities, like groceries or furniture. They are dealing with human beings and their lives. Mess up on a grocery delivery and you may ruin someone's dinner. Mess up on cosmetic surgery and you could ruin someone's life, or at least spoil their next few months.

The irony of this all is that cosmetic surgery is really *not* a gold mine at all. The revenue from Botox, collagen, laser surgery, and the like may look great on paper. But what many physicians—particularly those new to the field—overlook is that the overheads are high. When you factor in the cost of high-tech equipment, supplies, and the extra staff needed for cosmetic procedures, the bottom line may be little different from that of a doctor who's seeing general dermatology patients with acne, eczema and warts.

I believe it's vital that your cosmetic surgeon chose the field because it's what she enjoys doing and it fulfills her, not because she thinks it's a lucrative business venture. If your doctor has suddenly started to perform cosmetic surgery after several years in an unrelated field, ask why.

Avoid the Medical "Bait and Switch"

Gillian visited a well-known physician recommended by a friend to discuss Botox treatment of her crow's-feet and frown lines. She was told that

Caveat Emptor! Strategies for Choosing a Cosmetic Surgeon

207

she could, if she wished, have the procedure performed by this physician's partner, who was also board-certified, at another office closer to her home. Gillian jumped at the opportunity to shorten her travel time, and scheduled her Botox treatment with the partner.

The procedure improved her crow's-feet slightly but gave her a large, tender bruise around her left eye and drooping of her left eyelid for several weeks. It was only then that she discovered that the partner was indeed board-certified—but in OB/GYN! He'd had no experience of cosmetic surgery until he'd been hired to work in his current position.

Talk about a medical bait and switch. If you've checked out a doctor and are happy with him, make absolutely sure that he'll be the one who performs your procedure.

When Is It Okay for an Assistant to Perform Your Procedure?

What do you do when it's your doctor's assistant who treats you, rather than your doctor? This situation is appropriate for some procedures, if your doctor is around to provide medical supervision when needed. For instance, many medical assistants or aestheticians perform microdermabrasion, a painless polishing of the skin with fine crystals to improve wrinkles and discolorations. This noninvasive technique could be performed by any highly skilled assistant. If your doctor tells you that your microdermabrasion will be performed by his assistant, check out her training and experience just as you checked out your doctor's.

Many salons and spas now offer microdermabrasion alongside pedicures and massages. I strongly caution you against this. Although microdermabrasion is noninvasive, your skin can be permanently injured if the procedure is performed incorrectly. For instance, Vanessa was left with persistent discolorations on her cheeks after an overaggressive microdermabrasion by an unsupervised spa beautician inflamed her skin.

What's more, many of the microdermabrasion machines in spas and salons are less strong than machines designed for use only in a doctor's office, and they won't give you the same results. I perform my microdermabrasions with natural salt, rather than aluminum oxide, which is used in salons, spas, and most doctors' offices. Natural salt is more effective and totally safe.

There's been controversy recently over laser hair removal. I've personally seen patients like the ones you've probably read about who were burned and scarred after treatment by nonmedical personnel who were inadequately supervised. Maya is just one of them. A student in her mid-twenties, she experienced permanent scarring of her legs after her third session of laser hair removal at a salon in her local shopping mall.

Unfortunately, physicians of all specialties, and many salons, choose laser hair removal as their entrée into cosmetic surgery because they've been led to believe that it's a simple way of generating profits. It's easy to believe from the myriad of ads in the newspapers and magazines and on the radio that lasering away your unwanted hair is as easy as 1-2-3.

But nothing could be further from the truth. Thinking of laser hair removal as a formulaic, "point-and-shoot" process that can be turned over to assistants with minimal training and less supervision is a grave mistake. As with all lasers, one of the most important aspects of treatment is the correct strength. The amount of laser energy and the length of time for which it is delivered to your skin must be precisely adjusted, taking into account your hair and skin type and the location of your unwanted hair. For example, the bikini region of a woman with olive skin and black hair would require laser settings quite different from the upper lip of a fair-skinned woman with light brown hair.

Whoever designates the laser settings for your procedure must have an in-depth understanding of skin, hair, and the relevant laser physics. In my opinion, only a physician with extensive experience in cosmetic surgery is qualified to do this. You must have a medical history taken and a skin examination performed by this physician to determine whether you are a good candidate for the procedure.

Equally critical, whoever performs your laser hair removal must also know exactly what she's doing. A good hair laser technician is specifically certified to operate the machine she's using for your treatment, she's careful and methodical, and she doesn't hesitate to ask her supervising physician for advice when appropriate.

This supervision is the crux of the matter. An experienced, hands-on supervising physician should *always* be in the office when you're having your laser hair removal.

Caveat Emptor! Strategies for Choosing a Cosmetic Surgeon

209

I think some procedures should never be performed by anyone other than a trained physician because they are invasive procedures and, as such, require expert medical knowledge of your skin's anatomy. If you're told that your Botox, collagen, or fat injections will be performed by a nonphysician, ask why. There's no possible benefit from this to you as a patient—and a significant potential risk.

Avoid the "One Car in the Lot" Trap

Remember the story of Henry Ford's having said almost 100 years ago that the American public could have a Model T car in any color they liked, "so long as it's black?"

Today you'd never dream of buying a car from a salesman who told you that you needed a black car because that's all he had in his sales lot. But, much as I hate to compare doctors to car salesmen, patients make this kind of choice every day where their cosmetic surgery is concerned.

Lucy visited a local dermatologist for a skin checkup. The doctor, who advertised himself as an expert in collagen treatments, seemed less interested in Lucy's moles and her family history of skin cancer than in the lines around her mouth.

"He said that I needed collagen because my wrinkles were terrible and that I should have my first skin test right away," Lucy complained to me later. "He'd given me the skin test almost before I knew what he was doing!"

There is no such thing as a "collagen expert," any more than there's an expert in black cars—though it's easy to see why a physician who does no other cosmetic procedures might designate himself as such. Collagen treatment is easy to perform. If you know how to inject a patient's skin with numbing medication before removing a mole—and nearly all dermatologists do because it's a very basic skill—then you can inject someone's skin with collagen. The catch is, collagen treatment may be easy to do, but it's difficult to do *well*. That requires an artist's eye and an in-depth understanding of the aging process.

In Lucy's case, she never found out how good a "collagen expert" the doctor was because she didn't return to his office. Still, botched collagen—and botched Botox—treatments are depressingly frequent. That's why many patients are wary of changing physicians once they've found one who does a procedure the way they like it.

Anneliese is just one of my many patients who travel more than an hour each way to see me. After she moved, she tried out some local doctors for her thrice-yearly Botox injections, but in her words, "my husband told me to stop messing about with my face and just go back to you."

Don't ever allow yourself to fall into the "one car in the lot" trap. If the doctor you're consulting performs only a few cosmetic procedures, she may have a vested interest in pushing you into one of them, even if it can't give you what you want.

Look at what happened to Leigh, who wasted thousands of dollars on monthly collagen injections. Her doctor never told her that fat injections—which he couldn't perform—would give her better and longer-lasting improvement of her smile lines at a fraction of the cost.

You're better off finding a physician who can offer you a full range of options, so that he can objectively advise you about what will benefit you the most.

Avoid the New Doc on the Block

It's vitally important that you don't inadvertantly choose an entry-level cosmetic surgeon to treat you, as this increases your chances of a poor result. Fortunately, there's a pretty foolproof way to ensure that you don't find yourself in this nightmare situation: make sure that you get even the simplest procedure only from a physician who also performs the complex procedures.

There are four procedures that every doctor seems to be doing these days, regardless of whether she performs much cosmetic surgery. These procedures are relatively easy to do, so they're often presented to entry-level physicians as Cosmetic Surgery 101, even though they're actually difficult to do *well*. I mentioned one of these entry-level procedures earlier: collagen injections. The others are Botox, laser hair removal, and microdermabrasion.

These are the procedures that are advertised all over newspapers, magazines, and the radio. You'll see discount coupons, cut-rate prices,

Caveat Emptor! Strategies for Choosing a Cosmetic Surgeon

211

and promotional offers galore. The advertisements often give you no clue as to the qualifications and experience of the person treating you, nor do they tell you whether the procedures are performed in a doctor's office or in a salon.

In contrast, there are four procedures that are performed by relatively few physicians because they require greater skills. Physicians who do perform them tend to have a special interest and more extensive experience in cosmetic surgery. These advanced procedures are generally not advertised with scantily-clad women, special offers, or other gimmicks. They are fat injections, laser resurfacing of wrinkles, laser removal of spider veins and medium-depth chemical peels (also known as TCA peels).

The technique used to perform fat injections is an advanced version of what's used for collagen and Botox. Similarly, the skills required for laser resurfacing and laser removal of spider veins are an extension of those needed for laser hair removal. And the expertise needed for medium-depth chemical peels (also known as TCA peels) expands upon that required for microdermabrasion.

The rule is simple. You get an entry-level procedure only from a doctor who also has experience with the related advanced procedure. For example, I advise you to seek collagen injections from a physician who also performs fat injections. Any physician who's skilled enough to do fat injections is likely to do great collagen.

Don't Get Corralled into Surgery

I once worked in a dermatology group where the senior physician used to exhort her colleagues—and her staff—to "lasso that patient and bring her in for a procedure." This statement always conjured up in my mind the unfortunate image of women being corralled and herded into the operating room like mindless cattle.

If at any point during your consultation you feel that you are being pressured by a doctor or her staff into having a procedure performed, get up, say thank you, and simply walk away. Your doctor should be prepared to give you the facts and the options you need to make your own decision, without trying to push you into a corner. One of the most common complaints I hear from patients is that they feel uncomfortable with the "buy, buy, buy" atmosphere in some doctors' offices. Bridget was the most direct, telling me, "Every time I went in for my peel, they'd try to sell me another procedure. It was like going to the supermarket for a gallon of milk and being accosted by a salesman trying to persuade me that I needed everything else on the shelves too."

Make Sense of Those "Best Doctor" Lists

Most big cities have local magazines that regularly publish a list of "best doctors" in each medical specialty. So how useful are these lists for finding a good cosmetic surgeon?

Before you read these lists and act upon their advice, you need to

Know Your Docs

What's the difference between a dermatologist, a plastic surgeon and a cosmetic surgeon?

All board-certified physicians, including dermatologists and plastic surgeons, have earned medical degrees and then completed a 1-year internship in a general field such as internal medicine or surgery. After this, they proceed to residency and sometimes a fellowship—several years of specialized training in their respective fields. At the end of this training period, they are eligible to take exams in their specialty to become board-certified.

Dermatologist. Her training focuses exclusively on the skin and its associated structures—the hair, nails, and mouth. If she has a special interest in cosmetic dermatology, she performs skin rejuvenation procedures and often also liposuction since tumescent liposuction, now the gold standard method for doctors of all specialties, was developed and refined by dermatologists.

Plastic surgeon. His training includes reconstructive surgery—repairing birth defects and injuries due to disease or accidents—and also plastic surgery such as face-lift, rhinoplasty (nose job), and liposuction. A plastic surgeon with a special interest in cosmetic dermatology performs skin rejuvenation procedures.

Caveat Emptor! Strategies for Choosing a Cosmetic Surgeon

213

understand how they're created. I think the most reliable lists are based upon patients' experiences because they're most likely to be objective. Patients are randomly selected to complete a questionnaire indicating how satisfied they are with the doctors they have visited recently.

I think the least reliable lists are the ones based on surveys of physicians or on the opinions of the magazine staff themselves. There's no doubt that many of the doctors on these lists are indeed exceptional in their field. But keep in mind that this type of survey is highly subjective by definition. If you ask me which doctor I'd send my family members to, my decision is going to be based on a number of factors. Competence and bedside manner definitely factor into the equation, but so do personal friendships and professional relationships. These factors may

---

Cosmetic surgeon. Either a dermatologist or a plastic surgeon may call herself a cosmetic surgeon. And so may some ophthalmologists and otolaryngologists (ear, nose, and throat doctors), if they've developed a special interest in procedures that improve your appearance.

So how do you decide whom you should be seeing? You'll note that the pointers I've given you above are designed to help you find a good—hopefully, a great—cosmetic surgeon. I've specified individual characteristics that I believe are important for your doctor to have. But I haven't recommended doctors of a particular specialty for a particular procedure. I do think it's important that you avoid doctors

whose training is clearly unrelated to the field of cosmetic surgery, as with Gillian's Botox-botching OB/GYN and Lucy's general dermatologist turned "collagen expert". But if you've found a cosmetic surgeon with the appropriate training and experience, I believe your focus should be on determining whether he truly understands you and whether he is consummately skilled in performing the procedures you desire. His original field of specialization is a secondary consideration. If your doctor gives you the lips you've always dreamed of or smooths out your frown lines to perfection, does it really matter whether he's a plastic surgeon or a dermatologist?

not be at all relevant to you as a patient who's not my family member.

I had an interesting insight into a physician survey a few years ago when I was a member of a dermatology group practice. The founding member of the group had been in practice for more than 10 years and was rather put out that she'd never appeared on the "best doctor" list of a well-known local magazine. So she hired a public relations consultant, who advised her to establish a business relationship with her target magazine by placing glossy, high-profile advertisements in it. The consultant also ensured that I received one of the random questionnaires sent out to local physicians and told me that she would help me to complete it.

The strategy worked, and my physician colleague was featured on the next "best doctor" list of her target magazine. Unfortunately, she was not happy about the company she was in, stating that some of the other dermatologists who also made the list "didn't deserve" to be there.

My advice to you with any "best doctor" list is to integrate the information it gives you with what you hear by word of mouth and with your own impressions during a consultation.

Internet Physicians: On-line or Out of Line?

Everything's on-line these days, so it's hardly surprising that cosmetic surgeons have jumped on the bandwagon. Finding one who doesn't have a Web site is rare, but some surgeons have gone a step further and actually provide you with price quotes for procedures via the Internet, even if you've never met them in person.

I don't recommend that you select your physician on-line. The patients I've met who've dabbled in this method seem to know little about the doctors with whom they're communicating. Take Joy, who came to my office, waving a price printout for a chemical peel from a doctor who'd never seen her face and whose name she couldn't even remember.

Going with the lowest price quote for a given procedure may be a good strategy if you're buying a new car, but not if you're contemplating cosmetic surgery. I think you should seek a doctor whose experience you trust and with whom you have a good rapport. You can do this only if you meet her face-to-face. As I'll discuss below, your budget is certainly one of the considerations, but it shouldn't drive your selection process.

Caveat Emptor! Strategies for Choosing a Cosmetic Surgeon

215

Do You Get What You Pay For?

The answer to this question is yes and no. The key is to know what the approximate going rate for a procedure is. You can get this information by asking friends what they paid. You can also get it sometimes by calling doctors' offices, although many doctors are understandably reluctant to quote generic prices on the phone before they've seen you because the prices may not be relevant to you as an individual. However, you should be able to get some kind of ballpark cost over the phone for procedures like Botox treatment of your frown lines or laser hair removal on your upper lip.

The fees of most cosmetic surgeons for a given procedure in a given locality fall within a fairly well-defined range. They're based partly on the actual cost of the equipment for the procedure; for instance, Botox and collagen are expensive commodities, and most lasers cost tens or hundreds of thousands of dollars. And fees are also based partly on the physician's time and the skill needed for the procedure.

You'll note that I mentioned locality in this discussion of fees. Where you have your treatment can significantly affect how much you pay. Get your frown lines erased with Botox in Manhattan, and you'll likely pay two to three times more than you would for the same procedure in the Midwest or even where I practice, in suburban Maryland and Virginia. To some extent, this difference is justifiable: higher fees are based on the higher overhead it takes to run a doctor's office in a pricey locale. But to some extent, fees are simply based on what patients are prepared to pay. You can't do much about this, unless you're prepared to fly around America for the best deals.

Alarm bells should go off in your head if the surgeon you're consulting charges much more than the average—or much less. Either situation can indicate that the doctor doesn't perform this procedure frequently. If you find a really rock-bottom price, check the doctor's qualifications and experience all the more thoroughly. And when you're checking different offices' fees, make sure you know who will actually be treating you, so you are comparing apples with apples. It obviously costs less to have a nurse inject your wrinkles with collagen than to have a doctor do it.

Look for That Magic Touch

When patients tell me I'm a magician, they may think they're simply paying me a nice compliment. But in fact they're doing more than that. While I know great cosmetic surgery takes experience, competence, and good technology, experience tells me it also takes an artist's eye, consummate skill, and an indefinable flair—which is why I'm so grateful for my patients' praise.

I think I can best define the magic touch by telling you what it's *not*. A few years ago at a medical meeting, I overheard the conversation of two physicians who had just entered the field of cosmetic surgery.

"Collagen and Botox are so easy," one said to the other. "You put collagen in the wrinkles, and you put Botox between the wrinkles."

From a purely mechanistic point of view, this statement is not inaccurate. But mechanical collagen and Botox injections can never yield great results. The magic touch is what raises your procedure above a purely mechanistic level and what raises your results above the ordinary to almost mystical heights.

The magic touch is hard to find, but it's the Holy Grail of cosmetic surgery. It's not in the yellow pages, the newspaper ads, or even the "best doctor" lists, but you may find it through word-of-mouth recommendations or simple observation of another woman's results. If you're fortunate enough to find a doctor who has it, I advise you to hang on to her.

Perhaps my patient Adrienne said it the best: "Doctor, you see what I want before I even know it myself."

chapter twelve

Medical Solutions to Ten Cosmetic Curses

*Any sufficiently advanced technology is
indistinguishable from magic.*

—**Arthur C. Clarke**

hen I'm in my office, I often think of my favorite childhood story, *The Rose Geranium,* about a woman who received a beautiful flowering plant as a gift from a neighbor. When she placed the plant on her kitchen table, she was struck by how much nicer it would look if the table looked better. So she repainted the table. Of course, then the chairs didn't look so great, so she had to paint them too. Although the table and chairs looked wonderful, they really made the windows look shabby, but cleaning and some new curtains took care of that. And so on it went, until the woman's family came home to find the whole house made over and freshly baked cookies waiting for them on the kitchen table.

Many of my patients' makeovers are also jump-started by the first procedure—which is *their* rose geranium—and happen one step at a time. The advantage of this progression is that it gives my patients and me an opportunity to develop the rapport and mutual understanding we need

(continued on page 221)

Chemical peels and Laser resurfacing

Both of these methods work in the same manner: by removing layers of your skin. Where chemical peels and laser resurfacing differ is in how many layers of skin they remove. This determines the results you get from these procedures and how long it takes for your skin to heal.

Light chemical peels are performed by applying glycolic acid, another alpha hydroxy acid, or a beta hydroxy acid like salicylic acid to the skin. The peeling solution is left on the skin for a few minutes and then rinsed off with water. Cool compresses are then applied to soothe the skin. A light chemical peel removes the uppermost layers of your epidermis, which contain dead cells filled with keratin. The mild tingling or burning sensation you feel during the peel can be relieved by fanning your face during the procedure. Afterwards, your skin may feel warm, as if it is mildly sunburned, and look slightly pink. You can apply makeup and return to your normal activities immediately. The pinkness fades within a day or two.

A series of about four to seven peels spaced 1 to 3 weeks apart will gradually make your skin smoother and firmer and fade discolorations. Many patients subsequently choose to have maintenance peels a few times a year. I mentioned the debate over buffering of glycolic acid in chapter 9. I prefer minimally buffered, high acidity glycolic acid for chemical peels, just as I do for my patients' at-home skin regimens, as I've found it to be more effective. Light chemical peels usually cost about $100 to $150 per session. Some offices offer discount packages.

Medium chemical peels penetrate the skin more deeply, removing more layers of skin and stimulating the production of collagen and elastic tissue in the dermis. The traditional method is to apply a solution of trichloroacetic acid (TCA) to the skin and to leave it on for a few minutes until the skin has a white frosted appearance. The solution is washed off with water, cool compresses are applied and then the skin is covered with Vaseline or a similar soothing ointment. During a medium peel, you will experience mild to moderate stinging or burning and this may persist more mildly while your skin is healing after the peel. I usually treat the face in sections, rather than all at once, to minimize discomfort during the procedure.

I perform more medium peels these days using a TCA cream instead of a solution. I've found that this new technique, marketed by ICN Pharmaceuticals under the brand name, Accupeel, gives better results because the cream coats and penetrates the skin more evenly than the solution does. Patients usually have only 3 to 5 days of skin pinkness and flaking after an Accupeel, compared to 5 to 7 days with TCA solution of the equivalent strength. Any residual pinkness after the skin is healed tends to fade faster too. One or two medium chemical peels will significantly fade wrinkles, discolorations and some scars and tighten loose skin, especially around the eyes and the jawline. I also use the Accupeel to rejuvenate the neck, chest, back and hands.

The price of a medium chemical peel varies, but it is generally in the range of $600 to $2000 for treatment of the whole face.

Laser resurfacing is now the treatment of choice for skin rejuvenation beyond what can be achieved with medium chemical peels. A highly focused laser beam is directed onto the skin to vaporize its upper layers. The depth of skin vaporization can be exactly controlled by expert adjustment of the laser power and beam pattern. Discomfort during the procedure is prevented with numbing creams and local anesthetic shots and often with light sedation too. After laser resurfacing of the face, which takes about an hour, patients look and feel as if they have had a significant sunburn. Cool compresses and Vaseline or similar ointments soothe the treated skin and speed healing.

The older carbon dioxide (CO_2) lasers are very effective in stimulating formation of new collagen in the dermis but the skin remains red and raw-looking for about 2 weeks after treatment. It takes a further 2 to 6 months for pinkness of the healed skin to fade completely; meanwhile, this pinkness can be concealed quite well with makeup. Newer techniques of laser resurfacing have greatly shortened this recovery time without sacrificing results. Like many cosmetic surgeons, I now combine the CO_2 laser with the newer Erbium:YAG laser. This shortens healing time after treatment of the face to only 5 to 7 days; and subsequent skin pinkness

(continued)

Chemical peels and Laser resurfacing *(cont.)*

usually fades within 2 weeks to 2 months. It also allows me to individualize treatment much more precisely for a patient's aging pattern and skin type. I can treat skins of all colors, even darker skins which would be at risk of long-term discoloration from the CO_2 laser alone, or even from medium chemical peeling. I also use the Erbium:YAG laser to treat non-facial areas such as the neck, chest, back, arms, hands and legs.

Although laser resurfacing may sound like a rather involved process, many women will readily testify that laser resurfacing is well worth the effort, if it's performed well. The laser beam strongly stimulates the skin to produce large amounts of new collagen. This results in dramatic improvement in wrinkles, scars and loose skin, in addition to the fading of discolorations due to skin vaporization. Laser resurfacing is the ultimate in scar-free skin rejuvenation and it can take a decade or more off a patient's face. Treatment of the whole face costs about $4000 to $7000, depending on whether or not sedation is used.

Deep chemical peeling is mostly used by physicians who don't perform laser resurfacing. In experienced hands, the procedure is about as effective as CO_2 laser resurfacing but it carries the risk of heart or kidney problems. Patients' hearts must be constantly monitored during the peeling. Moreover, the phenol solution that is applied to the skin can cause scarring or permanent chalky-white discoloration of the skin. I don't use this method, as it offers no advantages, and significant disadvantages, over laser resurfacing. It should never be used on skin of color.

Dermabrasion (not to be confused with microdermabrasion) is a method of deep skin sanding using a rotating wire brush or wheel. Like deep chemical peeling, it produces good results in experienced hands but it carries the same risk of skin scarring or discoloration. It has also been largely supplanted by laser resurfacing.

Coblation is a recently introduced method of vaporizing surface skin layers with electrical energy. It can be used in skin of all types to improve mild to moderate aging changes and sun damage but it does not tighten the skin or improve deep wrinkles like CO_2 or combined CO_2/Erbium laser resurfacing.

to achieve the best results. Some women will always walk through the door knowing exactly what they want—like Cynthia, who requested the same type of lip enhancement I'd done for her friend with fat injections.

More commonly, my patients know they need a change but are hazy on what that change should be. As Cassie, a travel agent in her mid-forties, told me, "It's all so confusing; you go see a doctor and they tell you this is what you need to do, and they send you off to book an appointment. But you never get a clear idea of why they chose that treatment or whether there are any alternatives."

Finding the Right Solutions

I want you to know that there are *always* alternatives. Any problem has a number of solutions. I think it's vital for any woman to be an active partner in selecting the solution that will work for her. With the recent flood of media stories about new, potentially revolutionary cosmetic surgeries, I can understand that you may be bewildered by all the options available today. In this chapter, I want to steer you through the jargon and the hype. I'll tell you about the true medical breakthroughs—and the empty promises.

As you read on, keep one thing in mind. Brilliant technology alone is not a guarantee of a good outcome. You'll achieve the best results only if your doctor is prepared to sit down, talk to you, and get to know you as a person, not just as a name and a medical chart. I can look at your face for a couple of minutes and reel off the three procedures that will make the most difference to your appearance. But it takes longer to figure out the right procedures for *you* because that depends not only on what I think but also on what you want.

One consideration is your daily routine and whether or not you can take time out from it while your skin heals after a procedure. The doctor Cassie saw before me recommended that she have laser resurfacing of her whole face. From a technical point of view, this was the "right" procedure: It would certainly improve her wrinkles and sunspots significantly. But from Cassie's personal viewpoint, it was all wrong. She simply could not manage a week or two with a red, Vaseline-coated face.

"This is the busiest travel time of the year," she explained to me, "and there's nobody who can cover for me in the office."

You must also consider what makes you feel comfortable. If this is your first foray into cosmetic surgery, you may want to start light, with a procedure that doesn't feel too invasive to you. Cassie was eager to rejuvenate her face, but she had some misgivings. "I've never had any surgery in my life, apart from childbirth. Doing my whole face seems a bit drastic," she said.

In the end, we found a compromise so that Cassie could have her treatment over a holiday weekend without missing any office time. I lasered away her worst wrinkles, which were around her eyes, and I chemically peeled the rest of her face. Cassie went back to work wearing a little camouflage makeup to cover her facial pinkness for a day or two and dark glasses for a couple more days while the redness around her eyes subsided.

This arrangement not only fitted Cassie's schedule; it also felt less invasive to her and cost about half as much as laser resurfacing of her whole face. She was thrilled at the compliments she received from clients and coworkers afterward and even reported a business benefit from her treatment.

"My clients tell me I look really fresh and relaxed and ask me to recommend a vacation that will give them the same look," she giggled. "I should just tell them to hang out in your office for a week!"

What Questions Should You Ask about a Procedure You're Considering?

Some questions are obvious. You'll want to know how long the procedure will take, whether you'll need someone to drive you home afterward, and how much recovery time to expect. Don't be afraid to ask if you'll have any discomfort during or after the procedure and how you'll look immediately afterward. Find out how you will contact your doctor if you have questions or concerns after you've gone home.

Some of the procedures I'll be discussing require local anesthesia—numbing medication applied to or injected into your skin. Your doctor might recommend sedation for your comfort during two procedures, laser resurfacing and liposuction. If he does, find out how this will be administered. I feel that sedation via an intravenous line is safer because it can be more precisely controlled than medication given to you by mouth or by intramuscular injection. Make sure that a board-certified anesthesiologist will be monitoring your sedation with the appropriate equipment, whether it's in your doctor's office or in an outpatient surgical center. Your surgeon should be totally focused on your procedure, not distracted by your sedation. And the anesthesiologist who's monitoring your sedation should be totally focused on *his* job.

Understanding Your Pattern of Aging

At some point, every woman looks in the mirror and sees her mother looking back at her. Or, if not her mother, some other family member. I see this clearly when I look at my 8-year-old daughter. She has the same intense frown when she's reading that her grandmother—my mother— does, and no doubt she's destined to acquire the same furrow between her eyebrows.

I've asked you to step away from the notion that separate "intrinsic" and "extrinsic" factors determine how fast you age. It's an oversimplification because, in reality, many of these factors are interrelated and have both internal and external facets. More important from our point of view, the intrinsic factors are held to be inherited and uncontrollable. This encourages you to feel powerless about the aging process.

Where I do want you to factor in heredity is when you're considering your *pattern* of aging. Your lifestyle certainly affects your pattern, as well as your rate, of aging (think of smoker's lines around the mouth, or the freckles and discolorations on the cheeks that excess sun exposure produces). But to a large extent, the *way* you age is predestined.

First, consider your facial expressions. If you have your mother's smile or, like my daughter, your grandmother's frown, the chances are you'll eventually develop her smile or frown lines too. I find it fascinating to watch faces and see how close a correlation there is between how they express emotions and where they form wrinkles and creases.

Next consider your skin's elasticity, which determines how easily wrinkles will settle on your face and how late in life your eyelids and jawline will retain their tautness. Sun exposure and smoking profoundly impact your skin's elasticity. But we all start from a certain baseline of elasticity, and that's inherited. In general, darker skin has greater elasticity, and it tends to age by freckling rather than by sagging.

Now think of your bone structure. If you're born with high cheekbones, your eyes will probably survive the aging process fairly well, unless you damage your skin's support system through your lifestyle. Where you'll start to see aging is in the lower part of your face, as insidiously deepening smile lines and thinning of your cheeks. Conversely, your eyes and your jawline will suffer more if your cheekbones are lower.

Finally, consider your body weight. If you're slim, your jowls will tend to become looser, and your face more gaunt, with time. The plumper you are, the more likely you are to develop a double chin and puffy cheeks.

With these factors in mind, let's look at the basic patterns of aging and how they can be offset.

1. Your Forehead

Years of frowning or raising your eyebrows cause the forehead ridging known commonly as worry lines. Decreasing skin elasticity compounds this by sinking and flattening your eyebrows so that they lie closer to your eyelids. The eyebrows of a woman in her twenties have a graceful and feminine arch. But look at the brows of a 45-year-old, and more than likely you'll see that her arches have fallen and have a more masculine appearance.

A few injections of Botox relax the overactive muscles just beneath your skin and smooth out the lines. An innovative use of Botox is to actually raise your eyebrows—the so-called nonsurgical, or chemical, brow lift.

Botox has been high-profile news recently, and many women are fearful of it because of the reports they've read or heard. For instance Leslie, a 40-something realtor, told me wistfully, "I'd love to have Botox. But I don't want my face frozen so I can't show any emotions!"

Overtreatment with Botox prevents you from using your overactive muscles at all, and it will certainly give you that masklike, "deer caught in the headlights" expression you've probably seen on the faces of some women in the media. This blank look is a surefire giveaway that they've had Botox. But treatment with just the right amount of Botox in the right places weakens the overactive muscles in a controlled manner, smoothing out wrinkles while retaining your normal facial expressions. Skilled, professional eyebrow shaping to restore your feminine arches is the perfect complement to Botox treatment.

Leslie got rid of her frown and worry lines but could still raise her eyebrows and bring them together naturally. I also used Botox to lift her eyebrows subtly, and Mirvia then reshaped her eyebrows. Leslie had been brushing her auburn bangs over her forehead to hide the lines, but now she could sweep them up, giving her a more youthful look that emphasized her chiseled cheekbones and wide-set green eyes.

"Nobody has any idea I had Botox unless I tell them," Leslie reported gleefully. "But I'm getting loads of compliments on my new hairstyle and my skin!"

For more advanced forehead aging, surgical brow lifting is the solution. Whatever the method used to restore your eyebrow arches, there's one mistake you must not make. Run your finger over the contours of your eye socket, the bony depression in which your eyeballs are set. You'll feel a curved, slightly raised line of bone above your eyelids, where your eye socket joins the bone of your forehead. This raised line is medically known as the supraorbital ridge.

Elevate your eyebrows so that their highest point reaches this ridge when your face is relaxed, and they'll look great. But it is absolutely vital that your eyebrows not be raised above this ridge. Otherwise, you're going to be walking around with a telltale—and very unflattering—look of permanent surprise.

In certain social circles, this is all too common. My patient Hannah vividly described a high-society wedding she attended where "all the women had their eyebrows halfway up their foreheads" and thanked me (and the heavens) profusely for her own natural-looking Botox treatment

Botox and Other Muscle Relaxers

Botox is the brand name for purified botulinum toxin type A. It's injected in minute quantities into overactive facial muscles that lie just beneath your skin to relax them. Depending on where and how the Botox is injected, it will smooth out frown lines between your eyebrows, worry lines on your forehead, or crow's-feet around your eyes. It can also relax lines on your neck. The FDA (Food and Drug Administration) has officially approved Botox for the treatment of frown lines.

I've also used Botox to correct medical problems. For instance, Kate's surgery to remove a skin cancer left one of her eyebrows lower than the other, making her face look lopsided. I was able to even out her eyebrows quickly and safely with a couple of Botox shots.

Botox works by seeking out and binding to nerve endings, preventing them from overactivating your muscles. It's been used safely for more than 20 years to treat "lazy eye" in children and other eye problems in adults. Its wrinkle-banishing powers were discovered by accident during these medical treatments. It's now used for a myriad of other purposes, including migraine headaches and excessive sweating.

Injecting a minute amount of Botox into specific muscles is completely safe in healthy patients and carries no risk of the disease botulism, which is caused by eating food contaminated with much larger quantities of botulinum toxin. It's worth noting that some of our most effective and popular medications— including aspirin and Tylenol—are in fact poisons when taken in larger quantities than we use for treatment.

The injections usually take no more than a few minutes in total, and eyebrow shaping. Again, I'm sure you've seen this look on several of our more mature movie stars, and some younger ones too. A recent study showed that most women do end up with their eyebrows undesirably high after a surgical brow lift, presumably despite their surgeons' best intentions. I can't emphasize to you enough how important it is to discuss your aims with your surgeon or eyebrow shaper before she begins her work.

and each stings mildly for a fraction of a second. If you're worried about discomfort, you can use numbing cream before the procedure. The results take 1 to 7 days to appear fully. Immediately after treatment, you may have small red needle marks resembling tiny bee stings at the injection sites. You can cover these with makeup right away, and they fade within the next few days.

More rarely, you may get a small bruise for a few days at one or more of the injection sites. And, rarest of all, you may get drooping of an eyelid or eyebrow for a few days to a week or two. Other rare but reported temporary side effects include dry or watering eyes, headache, and sensitivity to light.

Expect your first Botox treatment to last 3 to 6 months, after which your wrinkles will reappear as they were. I've found that the wrinkles stay away longer in some patients who have Botox regularly; the mus-cles get retrained so that they're no longer so hyperactive.

How much your Botox treatment costs depends on where you live. But in general you'll pay a few hundred dollars for treatment of each area.

Other wrinkle relaxers include **Dysport**, a European version of Botox, and **Myobloc**, which is purified botulinum toxin B, a variant on Botox. Myobloc has been touted for use in patients who become resistant to Botox because they develop antibodies to it. I've personally never had a patient with resistance, but it's been reported in a few patients who have had large amounts of Botox injected into their necks. Like Botox, Myobloc relaxes wrinkles for 3 to 6 months, but the injections are more painful. Myobloc's biggest market may be physicians who perform only the occasional treatment because once it's opened, it can be stored in the refrigerator for much longer than Botox.

2. Your Eyelids

Sagging and bagging of your eyelids, and dark shadows under your eyes, can be fixed with chemical peeling or laser resurfacing. If you have very loose skin or prominent fatty pouches under your eyes, you may also need a blepharoplasty—an "eyelid job" in common parlance—to remove them.

Facial Fillers: Collagen

Fillers are substances that are injected into your skin to soften your wrinkles, smooth out pitted scars or enhance your lips. I generally stick to two fillers in my office—collagen and fat—as I've found them to be safe and extremely effective. (See "Facial Fillers: Human Fat" on page 230 for more information on fat injections.)

The collagen that's most commonly used in cosmetic surgery is purified from cows' skin and known as **bovine collagen**. Zyderm I is quite thin and used for fine lines, hollows under the eyes and shallow scars. Zyderm II is thicker and effective for deeper lines and scars. Zyplast is thickest and the collagen of choice for deep furrows and scars, and for lip enhancement.

Approved by the FDA for filling in scars and wrinkles, bovine collagen is very similar in structure to the collagen that gives support and resilience to the human dermis. On average, about three people in 100 are allergic to bovine collagen or to the anesthetic lidocaine, with which it's mixed. These people should not receive bovine collagen— nor should people who are allergic to beef—because they would develop red welts or bumps at the sites of injection. If you have lupus, rheumatoid arthritis, scleroderma or another connective tissue disease, you should avoid collagen injections, because you may be more likely to have significant allergic reactions.

If you're interested in bovine collagen treatment, two skin tests spaced at least 2 weeks apart could tell you whether or not you're allergic. During each test, a small amount of collagen is injected into the skin of your forearm; if you don't react, you're almost certainly not allergic.

Collagen injections usually take only a matter of minutes, but the results are quite dramatic: You can instantly see that your wrinkles or scars are filled in, or that your lips are fuller.

The method you choose depends on the amount of recovery time you can manage and your budget. Laser resurfacing, combined with blepharoplasty if you need it, will give you the best result, but you'll have to allow 4 to 6 days of healing time even with the most advanced lasers. The healed skin may remain pink for a month or more after this, and you

In fact, the treated areas are sometimes a little over-full or puffy for a few days, until the collagen settles down.

Tiny red marks the size of pinpricks in the areas where the collagen was injected and mild pinkness in the treated areas will disappear within a few days. You may develop a small bruise at an injection site, although this is not very common. In both of these cases, a little makeup can help you get back to your life without interruption.

Your body gradually breaks down the injected collagen, so this treatment usually needs to be repeated three or four times a year. The exact time between treatments depends on the individual patient and the treated areas. Sometimes, the treatment can stimulate your body to produce its own collagen, which will prolong the effects. I've seen this happen for some patients' lips, in particular.

The cost of collagen treatment depends on the type and amount of collagen used. In general, treatment costs from a few hundred dollars to fill in shallow smile lines, crow's-feet or hollows under the eyes to over a thousand dollars to treat deep furrows around the mouth and also enhance your lips.

Autologen is collagen which is extracted from portions of your own skin that have been removed during a facelift, tummy tuck or other surgery. It's impossible to be allergic to Autologen, unlike bovine collagen, because it is your own collagen. However, you need quite large pieces of skin to extract enough collagen to fill typical facial wrinkles.

Isologen is produced by taking a few collagen-producing cells from a patient's own skin and growing them in a test tube. It is not yet known whether these living cells are capable of producing enough collagen to fill in the wrinkles into which they are injected.

CosmoDerm is produced in a similar manner from the donated foreskin of an infant.

must protect it from the sun—otherwise, it may stay pink longer or even develop discolorations.

That's what happened to Alison, an architect in her early fifties. We scheduled her laser resurfacing for January since she spent most of the summer outdoors. The procedure tightened her eyelids and smoothed her

Facial Fillers: Human Fat

In addition to collagen, the other filler that I rely on in my office is **human fat**, which gives a more lasting result than collagen; many of my patients achieve a long-term improvement for several years.

First, I inject numbing fluid into a small area of a patient's buttock or abdomen and then remove, or harvest, the fat gently and painlessly, using a pencil-thin hollow tube. This tube, known as a cannula, is inserted into the numbed area via a tiny incision, no more than one-quarter inch in length, which is barely noticeable after it heals. It takes about 30 to 40 minutes to harvest two or three tablespoons of fat—enough to treat the desired areas over several sessions. Removing this small amount of fat from the buttock or abdomen does not change its shape appreciably.

Different surgeons have different methods of treating the harvested fat. Some like to rinse it and spin it at high speed in a centrifuge to remove fluid and blood that is mixed with the fat. With the method I use, I don't need to centrifuge the fat, as it contains very little blood. I simply drain off the numbing fluid, rinsing the fat gently if necessary to remove any traces of blood. I prefer to treat the fat as gently as possible, as I feel this increases the chances that it will survive and give long-lasting results.

Fat can be used to soften furrows around your mouth, fill in gaunt cheeks or scars and enhance your lips. I also like to use fat to contour the chin or cheeks; I find it gives a much softer and more natural-looking result than can be obtained with chin or cheek implants. Fat injections are also a wonderful rejuvenator for hands that have become bony and veined due to fat loss with age. The injected fat makes hands

wrinkles beautifully. But I was quite concerned when she missed her follow-up appointment with me a week later, and absolutely horrified when she called me the next day from Aspen, where she was staying with her boyfriend.

"I'm sorry," she told me breathlessly over the phone. "It was a totally spontaneous thing; Michael was free unexpectedly and he wanted look and feel dramatically younger and smoother. (Patients are at no risk of allergic reactions to their own fat, so they do not require skin tests before the injections.)

The areas to be treated are first numbed with anesthetic cream and small local anesthetic shots. The needle used to inject fat is wider than that used for collagen, so that living fat cells are not damaged when they pass through the needle. The temporary red marks from fat injections are somewhat larger, but fewer than those from collagen injections. If bruising occurs, it is usually minor, but larger bruises can develop occasionally. Red needle marks and bruising can be covered with makeup immediately after the procedure and they usually fade within a week. The treated areas may be slightly swollen, bumpy or tender for a few days.

Some surgeons prefer to inject fat only on the same day that it is har-

vested from the patient. Others, including me, inject some fat on that day and then freeze the rest in sterile syringes. This allows patients to return for touch-up injections with thawed-out fat over the ensuing months, rather than having to go through repeated fat harvesting procedures, until they obtain their desired results. A recent study showed that patients preferred both the results and convenience of frozen fat over fresh fat for the treatment of aging hands.

I often find that patients' faces can be rejuvenated most effectively by using a combination of fat and collagen injections. Fat is soft and provides natural-looking and long-lasting contouring of wrinkles, skin hollows and lips. Collagen, which is firmer, can then be injected on top of the fat to fill in the last traces of wrinkles and scars, or to precisely define lip borders.

to go skiing. But I promise I won't go outside for a minute without my goggles."

Despite Alison's best efforts, the mountaintop sun was intense enough to give her patchy brown discoloration where I'd lasered her under her eyes. It took 2 months for it to fade completely.

Chemical peeling is your best bet if you want only 3 to 5 days of

(continued on page 235)

Facial Fillers: Other Options

The past few years were marked by the Botox boom, the high point being the FDA's approval of Botox for wrinkle relief. Now, the next few years seem destined to be hailed as the Age of Fillers. Even as the popular press continues its love affair with Botox, it increasingly embraces a plethora of cosmetic fillers, besides collagen and fat, that are now available or soon to become so. It's understandable that the media focus on what's hot and new but, at times, this leads to rather disingenuous reporting.

For instance, **Artefill,** a combination of bovine collagen with synthetic plastic beads, has been touted by the press as the "perfect" filler. Artefill is certainly one of the more promising new fillers; it's been used in other countries for a number of years under the name **Artecoll** and has recently been approved by the FDA for use in the United States. Both of its principal ingredients—bovine collagen and Plexiglas beads—have a long track record of medical safety. And patients who report that the improvement in their wrinkles seems to get better with time have a point: the tiny beads in Artefill/Artecoll are designed to stimulate ongoing formation of your body's own collagen to provide longer lasting results than can be achieved with bovine collagen alone.

But I don't need to remind you that nothing's perfect, do I? As increasing numbers of patients in Europe and Canada are treated with Artecoll, reports have started to emerge of side effects. The most significant of these is the formation of granulomas—persistent hard nodules—in treated areas. This seems to occur most commonly when Artecoll is used for lip enhancement. It should be noted that Artecoll has never been specifically approved for injection into the lips. This is what's known as an "off label" use of a filler that has been approved for injection into smile lines and other wrinkles, just as Botox is used "off-label" when it's used to treat crow's feet, because it's only been approved by the FDA for frown lines.

What of other fillers? I think **Restylane** also has a future in the rejuvenation armory. It is a non animal-derived version of the hyaluronic acid which is naturally present in the dermis of your skin where it provides support and structure. It's used in other countries and is being investigated by the FDA for use in the United States. **Hylaform gel** and **Perlane** are similar to Restylane and they are also used in other countries. Studies have suggested that Restylane lasts longer than bovine collagen when it is injected into smile lines.

Then there's liquid **silicone**, which gained notoriety decades ago for its serious side effects when injected into the skin, but is now being studied in a more purified form. The silicone resurgence is fueled by its promise as a cheap and permanent cosmetic filler. But its permanence could actually be a disadvantage; what once filled your wrinkles beautifully may develop into unsightly bulges with time. That's what happened to Shelly, who had silicone injected into her

forehead and smile lines by the Californian plastic surgeon for whom she worked in the 1970s—silicone's heyday. As she continued to age, the fat layer on her forehead thinned but the injected silicone stayed the same. Much to Shelly's distress, she developed permanent swellings of silicone on her forehead and has had to resort to regular cortisone shots to decrease the swellings temporarily. Bottom line, liquid silicone is not approved by the FDA for injection into the skin and no woman should contemplate wrinkle treatment with silicone until its safety is established beyond doubt.

I don't feel that other fillers offer any advantages, in either effectiveness or safety, over bovine collagen and human fat. **Alloderm, Cymetra, Dermalogen, Dermaplant** and **Fascian** are extracted from the skin of human cadavers. **Fibrel** consists of freeze-dried pig gelatin mixed with plasma from the patient's own blood.

Gore-Tex, Softform and **Ultra-Soft,** which are made of a pliable synthetic material, are threaded underneath wrinkles or lip borders to raise them up permanently. The re-

(continued)

Facial Fillers: Other Options (*cont.*)

sults are dramatic, but often not very natural.

Moreover, the implants can shift within the skin or even begin to poke out from it. Karina is one of my patients who's had problems with these implants. The Gore-Tex thread, which was embedded beneath one of her smile lines by another surgeon, shifted upward after a few years, so that it actually deepened and worsened the smile line it was originally intended to improve. It can be quite difficult to remove displaced implants due to the surrounding scarring. In Karina's case, I left the Gore-Tex in place, but injected fat below and around it to fill in her smile line, after gently breaking up the scar tissue with a broad-based needle. This procedure was quite challenging, but ultimately rewarding, as Karina was delighted with her results.

Don't let the media hype over fillers blind you to a couple of important facts. First, reports of Botox's demise in the wake of the filler revolution are greatly exaggerated. Neither Artefill nor any other filler can do what Botox does, which is to actually smooth out wrinkles caused by overactive muscles (these are known as dynamic wrinkles) rather than to merely fill them in. Second, there's no "perfect" filler for every face and I doubt there ever will be. I hope you understand by now that your face has its own individual pattern of aging which requires an individualized combination of treatments. Any cosmetic filler will only be as good as the hands of the cosmetic surgeon in which it rests.

down time. If properly performed, it will still give you good results, and, at a few hundred dollars, it's about one-third to one-quarter the cost of laser resurfacing. In either case, I find pretreatment with Botox very helpful. And Botox alone can work wonders for your crow's-feet.

If you can't manage any down time, then look at the CoolTouch or NLite laser. Either will improve your wrinkles over a series of sessions, and you'll have little more than mild pinkness for an hour or two each time. But they will not tighten your skin or remove discolorations the way that laser resurfacing or chemical peeling will. Collagen injections under your eyes can be helpful for dark circles.

3. Your Cheeks and Nose

Gauntness of your cheeks and deepening smile lines are best treated with injections of fat or collagen. Fat is your body's own natural filler, and it gives wonderful results if injected correctly. You may experience a little hardness or lumpiness in your cheeks for the first few days or weeks, but this will eventually soften and be totally undetectable. Fat is best used for recontouring in facial areas where you've lost fat with age. Collagen is firmer than fat, and I like to use it for fine sculpting.

I often achieve the best results by combining fat and collagen injections. Marianne's high Gallic cheekbones had always given her face a classically ethereal look that perfectly matched her petite frame. But as she entered her late fifties, she could not help but notice the changing contours of her face. And others noticed too.

"People keep telling me I look tired and asking if I've lost weight," she sighed.

The challenge with Marianne was to rejuvenate her without over-powering her delicate bone structure. A teaspoon too much fat or collagen in the wrong place would have rounded her face too much and detracted from her cheekbones. I filled in her cheeks and smile lines with fat and then placed a layer of collagen over the fat in her smile lines. The results were stunning and undetectable to anyone who was not in the know.

If your skin is hanging in loose folds, fillers are not enough, and

(continued on page 238)

Eyelid-lifts, Brow-lifts and Face-lifts

Blepharoplasty, known as an eyelid-lift, involves surgical removal of loose skin from the upper eyelid or from the lower eyelid which lies just below your eyes. In addition, fat pockets under the eyes are removed or repositioned and muscles may be tightened, improving droopy eyelids and bags under the eyes.

Younger patients who don't have much loose skin can take advantage of the newer method of transconjunctival blepharoplasty to remove their under-eye pouches. The surgical incision is concealed on the inside of the lower eyelids, which can shorten the recovery time. In older patients whose eyelids are loose, the incision for a lower eyelid blepharoplasty is made just below the eyelash line. The incision for upper lid blepharoplasty is placed in the natural fold of the upper eyelid. Blepharoplasty is performed using numbing eye drops and sedation and it takes about an hour to treat the upper and lower eyelids.

Bruising and swelling around the eyes usually subsides within two weeks and it can be covered by makeup after the first week, once any non-dissolvable stitches are removed. You can resume light daily activities and wearing contact lenses in a week to 10 days but you may have to refrain from strenuous activities for 2 weeks or more. Blepharoplasty can be combined with laser resurfacing on the same day for complete rejuvenation around the eyes with simultaneous recovery. The blepharoplasty takes care of the loose skin and fat pouches, while the laser resurfacing improves skin texture and discolorations. Blepharoplasty of the upper and lower eyelids usually costs a few thousand dollars. If your eyelids droop so much that your vision is impaired, this surgery may be covered, at least in part, by medical insurance.

Brow-lifting, or forehead-lifting, is traditionally performed by making a surgical incision along your scalp an inch or two above the hairline. Loose skin is then pulled upwards and stitched into place after the excess skin has been cut out, smoothing out deep furrows on the forehead and between the eyebrows and decreasing eyelid droop. Endoscopic brow lifting is a new, less invasive option for younger patients whose wrinkles are less deep. Several tiny incisions are made on the scalp, instead of one long incision, and small surgical instruments, including a fiber optic camera, are gently placed into these incisions. The surgeon releases the skin from any fibrous bands which are furrowing it and tightens the skin from within.

Your scalp may be bruised and swollen for a week or two after surgery and it may be numb for longer, perhaps even permanently. You can return to light daily activities after about 2 weeks but may have to wait up to 2 months before resuming strenuous activities. Brow-lifting takes 1 to 2 hours under sedation or general anesthesia and typically costs $3000 to $6000.

Face-lifting, or rhytidectomy, is an extension of the brow-lifting technique. The extent of the procedure varies, depending on whether the skin alone is tightened or whether the underlying muscle and fibrous tissue is too. Neck-lifting may also be combined with face-lifting. The surgical incisions are hidden as much as possible behind your hairline and ears and under your chin. A well-executed face-lift will tighten your skin and smooth out deep wrinkles around the eyes, on the cheeks, around the jawline and on the neck. The procedure takes about 2 to 5 hours under general anesthesia.

Your face and neck will be swollen and bruised for up to 2 months after surgery. And you may experience numbness of some areas for 6 months or longer and, occasionally, even permanently. Portions of the surgical scars may remain raised, red or tender for 6 months to a year. Face-lifting typically costs between $4000 and $10,000, depending on the extent of the procedure.

3. Your Cheeks and Nose *(cont.)*

you need to consider a face-lift, where your skin and its underlying muscles are surgically cut and pulled tight. But I urge you to consider—and discuss with your surgeon—combining your face-lift with fat or collagen injections in your cheeks. These injections have a softening effect and can prevent you from looking overtightened and obviously "done."

You have a variety of options for skin discolorations, and I often find that combining these works best. For instance, I laser-resurfaced Pam's face to remove the patches of brown discoloration that were a legacy of her childhood spent by the beach. During this procedure, I used another laser, the Diolite, to remove the sharply defined darker freckles and moles on her cheeks. The Diolite laser can also be combined with chemical peeling or with salt macrodermabrasion in the same way, so that different types of discoloration can be treated simultaneously. In Pam's case, the bonus from her laser treatment was that I also used it to remove the spider veins from her nose and cheeks.

4. Your Mouth

Very few women have the same mouth at 50 that they had when they were 25. But thinning, puckering, and downturning of your lips is such an insidious process that you may not actually be aware of these changes unless you scrutinize a photograph of yourself at a younger age.

What many women do notice, though, is that their lipstick doesn't stay put. Ursula, a teacher in her mid-forties, had actually stopped wearing it because "I just end up looking like I have a red mustache."

Of all the procedures I perform, lip enhancement is one of my favorites. It's instant gratification for me to be able to transform a face in just minutes. But Ursula was apprehensive because of the overdone lips she'd seen in movies and magazines.

"I don't want my lips to walk into the room before I do," she demurred.

I generally take lip enhancement slowly and in stages because so many women have similar fears. I reshaped Ursula's lips with fat injections in four sessions over a 3-month period, followed by a session of collagen injections. I first made her lips as symmetrical as possible and then recontoured their borders so that they turned outward slightly to give her a subtle pout. This eversion, as it's medically known, corrected the elongated distance between her nose and mouth and restored her "white line"—the thin, lighter-colored rim of skin immediately above her lips. When Ursula ran her finger from her nose down to her mouth, she could now feel a slight ridge where her skin ended and her lips began.

The overall effect was to restore Ursula's mouth to what it had been in her twenties. This happened so gradually that it was totally undetectable to an outside observer. Ursula was amused no end when friends kept telling her how beautiful she looked because of her new lipstick.

"They don't realize it's not my new lipstick; it's my new lips!" she said, laughing.

5. Your Jawline and Neck

Whether or not you develop jowls and a double chin depends to some extent on how much you weigh, but also on your genes. Invariably, every woman who walks into my office with these problems cites a family member from whom they're inherited them. For Miranda, a 38-year-old research scientist, it was her mother, and she brought me a photo of the two of them together to prove it.

"My face has never been slim," she told me. "But now I'm losing my neck completely, and I can't stand these chipmunk cheeks."

I love to look at Miranda's before and after photos. I removed the excess fat from her neck, jawline, and cheeks through three tiny incisions, each less than one-quarter inch long, that were hidden under her chin. I had warned Miranda to expect bruising and puffiness because I was liposuctioning her face as well as her neck. But she had hardly any and looked wonderful just 2 days after the procedure. Over the next 6 months, she looked better every time I saw her. Now her neck is long and graceful, and her cheeks and jawline perfectly set off her round blue eyes. She's given me permission to show her pictures to other patients, and some of them actually gasp when they see her transformation.

If the skin of your neck is hanging in folds, you may well need a neck lift, where, as with a face-lift, your skin and muscles are surgically cut and pulled tight. However, I see many women whose doctors have recommended this procedure but who in fact don't need it. Miranda was one; two surgeons had told her previously that liposuction without a neck lift would leave her with loose skin under her chin. But she was assiduous about wearing the postliposuction chin strap I recommended, and her skin recontoured itself perfectly after the procedure.

I've even found that skin that's likely to be a little loose after liposuction can be coaxed back into shape with laser resurfacing. I perform this the same day as the liposuction, and it has the added benefit of removing freckles and discolorations. The advantage of this treatment combination over a neck lift is that the recovery time is much shorter, and the tiny, hidden scars become almost imperceptible with time.

Spider veins and discolorations on your neck, as on your face, are due to sun damage. They can be treated effectively by combining laser resurfacing or chemical peeling with Diolite or a similar laser treatment.

6. Your Hands

One of the most common mistakes women make is to nurture their faces and neglect their hands because your hands can betray your age even when your face doesn't.

Dorothy, a motivational speaker in her late forties, was only too aware of the importance of fixing her hands as well as her face. They were on constant display at the seminars and workshops she conducted, and she was becoming increasingly self-conscious about their prominent veins and boniness. She was religious about sun protection, even going so far as to wear white cotton gloves when driving. But a childhood spent in Southern California had taken its toll, and she'd developed brown spots on the backs of her hands. I'd treated the sun damage on Dorothy's face and neck with laser resurfacing a year previously, and she'd been very pleased with the results. Now it was time to work on her hands.

Your hands, like your neck, often do best with a combination of procedures. I laser-resurfaced Dorothy's hands to tighten the skin and also treated them with the Diolite laser to fade the sunspots. Then I injected fat beneath the skin to cover the veins and boniness. She was delighted with how her hands looked afterward, and how they felt.

"Almost everyone I shake hands with comments on how soft and smooth my hands are!" she reported triumphantly.

7. Excess Hair

There's one secret about hair lasers that I want you to know. They all work, despite the ads touting one laser as being the only one for you. The challenge is to find the one that has the fewest side effects. If you're light-skinned and have dark hair, that's not too difficult. The issue for you is to make sure your doctor knows what he's doing and sets the laser correctly to target your hair as aggressively as possible.

But if you are of Mediterranean, Latin, Middle Eastern, Asian, or African ethnicity, you need to choose hair lasers carefully. Many will tend to inflame even the palest olive skin because their energy is absorbed not only by the pigment in the hair but also by the pigment in the skin. The resulting inflammation can lead to skin discoloration that can be annoyingly tenacious.

I've used a variety of hair lasers over the years and now stick with the one I've found to be best for all skin types. It's called the Apex, and it causes little skin inflammation because it precools the skin to a greater degree then other lasers. I can also adjust the time between laser beam pulses much more precisely than with other lasers. This timing allows your skin to recover fully from one pulse before it receives another, again decreasing the tendency for inflammation. Even my fair-skinned patients are better off because the Apex can also be used on them without skin precooling, allowing the removal of hair that persists with other hair lasers.

Laurie, a 22-year-old architecture student, had been through six sessions of laser hair removal at a salon before she'd come to see me. She was disappointed that she'd seen little reduction in the dark hair on her upper lip and chin. Since she was light-skinned, I was able to use the Apex without skin precooling, and she achieved excellent results.

Laser Hair Removal

All **hair lasers** work—your strategy should be to find the one that works for you without causing side effects. And, of course, to make sure that laser is in the right hands! All hair lasers target the pigment surrounding the base of your hair follicles; that's why they don't work on blond or white hair, which has no pigment. The laser energy is absorbed by the pigment, generating heat that damages the hair follicles and prevents them from producing hair. The key to successful laser hair removal is selectivity: the hair follicles should be damaged without significant damage to the surrounding skin.

This distinction is relatively easy for light-skinned patients with dark hair; the dramatic contrast between hair and skin makes selectivity a snap, even for the older lasers. Recent research on improving selectivity for patients with lighter hair or darker skins has led to newer lasers which precool the skin to minimize damage to it during treatment. Now some settings are so refined that the laser beam can pass harmlessly through the skin to reach its target hairs.

If you have a specific area—let's say, the upper lip—treated with a hair laser, it can only destroy those hairs that happen to be in the active growing stage of their life cycle at the time of treatment. On average, five treatment sessions spaced 3 to 6 weeks apart are needed to capture all unwanted hairs in this growing stage. The coarser and darker the hair, the more sessions it's likely to require. The hair falls out immediately after treatment with some lasers, whereas with others it can take a week or more.

During treatment, you will feel a series of pinprick-like sensations as the laser beam is applied to your skin. Precooling of the skin minimizes discomfort but many of my patients prefer to use numbing cream before treatment, especially for large,

8. Hair Loss

If you're between ages 30 and 50 and have started to notice diffuse thinning of your hair, you're not alone. This time can bring perimenopausal changes in your hormone levels and hair growth cycles. But it's vital that sensitive areas like the legs or bikini region. After treatment, your skin may be slightly pink for a few hours to a few days. Even with today's lasers, you should be prepared for the possibility of temporary skin redness or mild scabbing, if you have pigmented skin.

If you read laser hair removal advertisements, you'll find a recurring theme. Many hair lasers are described as "FDA approved for permanent hair reduction." What this means is that you may have some hair re-growth after completing a course of laser hair removal but it will tend to be lighter in color and finer in texture. In real terms, you'll no longer have that dark shadow over your lip or under your arms after successful laser hair removal. However, you may find yourself returning for further treatment months or years later. This is particularly true for stubborn hairs on the chin or upper lip, which seem to increase in number during times of hormonal

change, such as pregnancy, peri-menopause or menopause.

Despite these caveats, laser hair removal stacks up very favorably against electrolysis, the only other method of permanent hair removal, because it's much quicker and more comfortable. Only a few minutes per session for a few months are required to laser the upper lip or chin and about an hour for the entire legs. It usually takes several hours over a number of years to do this with electrolysis. And laser hair removal doesn't give your skin the tell-tale open-pored look that's a sure give-away of electrolysis—due to repeated insertion of the electrolysis treatment needle down the same hair follicles.

Laser hair removal at a qualified physician's office typically costs $200 to $250 per session for the upper lip or chin and more for larger areas. However, discount packages are usually available and you often receive significant additional discounts if you're treating more than one area at once.

you—and your doctor—don't fall into the trap of assuming that hormonal changes are the only reason for hair loss at this stage of your life. Otherwise, you may miss another reason that's staring you in the face.

That's what happened to Lydia. An attorney in her late thirties, she'd been told by her previous dermatologist that her widening part was age-related. He had suggested that she consider hair transplantation. At first sight, Lydia seemed to have no problems with her hair, which was stylishly pulled back into an elegant chignon. But a closer look told a different story. There were numerous short, broken hairs on the crown and the front of her scalp. When I examined her hairline, I found that it had receded at her temples. And I had a diagnosis: traction alopecia, the medical term for hair loss due to excessive pulling on the roots.

Lydia had inherited her naturally curly hair from her father. To achieve the smooth, sleek style she favored for work, she had to blow-dry her hair on high heat and then run a hot straightening iron over it several times. After years of this routine, her hair was so severely heat-damaged that when I pulled gently on it, several strands broke off in my hand. I explained to Lydia that she must stop straightening her hair and pulling it back tightly from her face. Otherwise, she risked developing areas of permanent baldness.

At this stage, I was pretty sure I knew why Lydia was losing hair. But I still ran baseline blood tests to check for anemia, an overactive or underactive thyroid gland, and other conditions that could also be contributing to her hair loss. Real life is rarely as simple as the textbooks, and I've seen many women over the years who had multiple reasons for their hair loss.

When Lydia followed up with me a month later, I could see that she'd taken my advice to heart. Her hair had its natural curls, and although she'd still put it up, it was in a looser style. But there was one problem we had not foreseen.

"I love my new hairstyle, but my boss doesn't," Lydia sighed. "He thinks it makes me look less professional, and he's concerned that a judge or a client may feel the same way."

Fortunately for Lydia—and her hair—she won her next court case spectacularly, and that was the last she heard about the supposed impact of her hairstyle on her professional competence. Within 6 months, her hair was much less fragile and brittle and the breakage had stopped.

Hair transplantation was not the right treatment for Lydia. But it's definitely an option if your thinning hair is due to age. With this treatment, thick hairs from the back of your scalp are shifted to the thinning areas at the crown and front. This painstaking process usually takes several sessions. The transplanted hairs are usually retained well in their new location. But be aware that hair transplantation is not a permanent fix for

Hair Transplantation

Hair transplantation is performed by numbing the back of your scalp with local anesthetic shots, removing hair from this area and inserting them into areas where your hair is thinning. A variety of techniques can be used: single hairs, groups of hairs or even whole strips can be repositioned where they are needed. The best and most natural-looking results are obtained with a combination of techniques. The key is to avoid uniform rows or large clumps of hairs that look like a toothbrush or the hair on a doll's head. That's what happened to May, a thirty-seven year old graphics designer. She ended up having laser hair removal to get rid of a hair transplant that looked disfiguringly unnatural.

Scars in the area from which the hair is removed can be hidden by the surrounding hair; most women who experience hereditary hair loss tend not to thin too much at the back of their scalps. The areas to which the hair is transplanted may be tender, swollen or crusted for a few weeks to a few months after the procedure.

Keep in mind that hair transplantation is an ongoing process. You will probably need several sessions initially to correct moderate hair thinning. And you'll require further sessions to maintain results as your hair continues to thin. This can be expensive and time-consuming. One session of hair transplantation alone can take several hours and typically costs $3000 to $5000. However, hair loss can be so devastating for many women that they feel the time and expense are well worth it.

your problem. You will tend to lose more hair with time and require ongoing sessions of hair transplantation to maintain your results, which can be both time-consuming and costly.

9. Acne and Rosacea

"It's time!" Gretchen announced as she strode into the exam room. Indeed it was. It was 6 months to the day since Gretchen, a professional fundraiser in her early forties, had completed treatment with Accutane (a brand of isotretinoin) for the persistent, severe acne on her face and back. Now she was ready for the next step—to free herself of the scars.

Gretchen had sailed through her teenage years with barely a pimple. But her acne had begun insidiously around the time she'd turned 30. Her skin worsened in the ensuing years, and she first noticed acne cysts on her face after her second pregnancy, when she was 36. These cysts were hard, red, tender, and extremely embarrassing for Gretchen, whose job required her to attend social functions several times a month. When the cysts eventually healed, they left persistent dark spots. To make matters worse, she started to develop rosacea too, and the stress of a big event frequently left her cheeks and nose flushed and flaming red.

Gretchen often came to see me before a big event so that I could inject a mild cortisone into the cysts. This treatment would magically flatten them within a day or two. Cortisone is a great remedy for a woman who has the occasional cyst, but it was clearly inadequate for Gretchen. Her acne barely improved with antibiotic pills and lotions, and I discussed Accutane treatment with her on several occasions. In my experience, about 50 percent of patients are completely cured of their acne after taking a course of Accutane, a relative of vitamin A and the strongest acne medication available. At the very least, Accutane will always tame acne and make it more responsive to other treatments.

Gretchen relished the prospect of being rid of her acne for good, but she was concerned about the side effects that she might experience, particularly the possibility of liver inflammation. A couple of decades previously, she'd had a very unpleasant bout of hepatitis A while backpacking in Southeast Asia. She'd recovered fully once the viral illness had run its course, but it had left an indelible impression on her mind.

"I just have this incredible fear that I'm going to end up jaundiced again," she told me.

I've treated enough patients with Accutane to truly think of it as a miracle. Unless you or someone you're very close to has had severe acne, you cannot fully appreciate its devastating impact. Even if the acne eventually burns out, there's little escape from the lifelong, stigmatizing scarring. Accutane has transformed innumerable lives, saving patients—and their physicians—from situations of utter desperation.

Accutane has received some bad press recently, but I'm convinced of its safety if it's used as recommended. I'm rigorous about seeing patients regularly and checking the appropriate blood tests during their treatment course, which lasts about 5 months. And I've never had a single patient with a serious side effect that's affected her general health, even though I've taken a handful of patients off Accutane midcourse because their liver enzymes or blood fats became elevated. But, as I pointed out to Gretchen, they were not even remotely ill, and their blood tests went back to normal within a month or two. The only way Gretchen could become jaundiced and sick on Accutane was if her blood were not tested regularly—and I would never allow that to happen.

The turning point for Gretchen came when the cysts started appearing on her back.

"Now I feel terrible about even wearing an evening gown," she confessed to me on the eve of her 43rd birthday. "Let's just do it."

Gretchen's Accutane treatment was a resounding success, and the only side effects she experienced were dryness of her lips and face, which were easily controlled with noncomedogenic moisturizer and mild cortisone creams. With her acne gone, Gretchen was eager to tackle her scars. But that's when the waiting comes in because Accutane affects the way your skin heals while you're taking it and for some time afterward. If I treated Gretchen with laser resurfacing, chemical peeling, or other surgery as soon as she was done with the Accutane, there would have been a small but definite risk that she might develop disfiguring, raised scars.

Gretchen had literally been crossing off every day on her calendar, and when the 6-month time limit had elapsed, she was ready for action. I used a selection of the techniques in my armory for her. First, I cut out the deep, pitted scars on her cheeks and forehead and sewed her skin back together with stitches no thicker than human hairs. With a broad-based needle, I gently broke up the bands of fibrous scar tissue that bound down the wider, troughlike scars on her face. I then used the same needle to fill these loosened scars with Gretchen's own fat. The next step was to laser-resurface her whole face. Finally, I filled in with collagen the tiny pinpoint scars that remained.

I treated Gretchen in sessions extending over several weeks, using numbing cream to keep her comfortable during the procedures. Meanwhile, I was also working on her back. Her scarring here was more superficial, and I was able to fade it quite well with alternating sessions of salt macrodermabrasion and glycolic acid chemical peels.

I was worried that Gretchen might be disappointed with the results.

Microdermabrasion and Macrodermabrasion

You've probably heard about *microdermabrasion* under one of its many brand names, which include the Power Peel, Parisian Peel and the MegaPeel. Microdermabrasion was riding the crest of the "lunchtime procedure" wave a few years ago, a pain-free procedure that promised to restore your skin's youthful glow with little or no recovery time. And, indeed, it's made many women—and men—extremely happy.

The simple procedure can be used successfully on skin of all colors. Tiny aluminum oxide crystals flow from a machine into a hand piece and onto the skin, to polish and gently exfoliate it. In a variant of classical microdermabrasion, no crystals are used but a diamond-studded hand piece polishes the skin instead.

Treating the entire face takes about 20 or 30 minutes. The neck, chest, back and just about any other skin area can also be treated. Some diehard aficionados even swear by total body microdermabrasion, for baby-soft skin all over. After treatment, your skin may be slightly pink or flushed, usually for an hour or two but occasionally overnight. You can apply makeup immediately after the procedure.

I've now moved from microdermabrasion to a newer method that I—and my patients—have found to be more effective. The skin is polished with natural salt crystals instead of aluminum oxide—a procedure known as **macrodermabrasion**, or "salt peeling."

I first tried out this procedure a few years ago, on three patients who had previously had several sessions of microdermabrasion and were pleased with it. I was struck by the fact that all of them called me afterwards to report better results with

Although her skin was immeasurably improved, it was not—and could never be—perfect. But my worries evaporated the day that she came to see me, carrying a glossy boutique shopping bag.

"See this?" she announced as she pulled an impossibly glamorous backless crimson silk sheath from the bag. "Now I'm really going to paint the town red!"

the salt peeling. And I was even more impressed when I saw for myself how their skin texture, prominent pores, discolorations, acne and superficial scarring improved with further salt peels. Another patient, Cecilia, minced no words when she told me, "Four sessions of salt peeling have done more for my skin than four years of microdermabrasion."

Salt peeling is simply an updated and more potent version of the salt scrubs whose beneficial effects upon the skin have been known since antiquity. My original motivation in substituting salt crystals for aluminum oxide was my general philosophy of holistic skin care and my desire to use as many natural therapies as possible. It was a surprise and a delight to me that the results of salt peeling were so much better too. I think one reason for this is that salt, unlike aluminum oxide, dissolves in water and may be able to hold moisture effectively within the upper layers of the skin, so that it feels markedly softer and smoother after treatment. Additionally, high concentrations of salt have a powerful antibacterial effect—that's why pickling in salt is an effective method of preserving food. This may be why salt peeling often has such a profound effect upon acne, which is characterized by an overgrowth of the skin's own resident bacteria.

Whether you choose to have microdermabrasion or macrodermabrasion, you'll require several sessions of treatment, usually spaced 1 to 3 weeks apart, to achieve the best results. On average, my patients have between four and seven sessions. Some opt for maintenance treatments a few times a year to maintain their glow and stave off the effects of time. The cost per session varies quite markedly, depending on your locality. As a general rule, treatment of your face in a physician's office will cost $150 or more per session. Many offices offer discount packages if you purchase several sessions in advance.

10. Prominent Pores

When it comes to pores, most women will tell you that size really does matter. Which is why you may be shocked to learn that your pores—the openings through which your hairs reach your skin's surface—actually stay the same size throughout your life. What *does* change is their prominence.

(continued on page 253)

Liposuction

Of all cosmetic surgery procedures, **liposuction** is the target of the most controversy. Liposuction is becoming increasingly popular. According to the American Society for Aesthetic Plastic Surgery (ASAPS), the number of liposuction procedures performed annually in 2001 (385,390) was more than double the number performed in 1997 (176,863).

Yet, despite this increasing demand, many women are haunted by media-driven images of liposuction as dangerous and ineffective. They remember the magazine cover stories that tell of death or serious disability after liposuction; or movies such as *Clueless*, in which the heroine's mother is said to have died during a routine liposuction. And then there are the interviews with women who assert that liposuction didn't do a thing for them because "the fat all came back."

To understand the debate over the safety and effectiveness of liposuction, you must first understand the procedure itself. Liposuction was developed in France and introduced to the United States in 1982. It was originally performed under general anesthesia in a hospital setting, until a dermatologist, Dr. Jeffrey Klein, developed the tumescent liposuction technique in 1987 with the aim of maximizing patient safety. Tumescent liposuction allows stubborn areas of fat to be removed in an outpatient setting, with little discomfort and quick recovery. This is now the gold standard in facial and body contouring and has been adopted by physicians of other specialties.

In liposuction of the face and neck, anesthetic fluid is injected just beneath the skin to numb the treated areas. The unwanted fat is then gently sucked out through a small hollow tube or cannula. This cannula is inserted into a single tiny incision, concealed under the chin, which heals well and becomes almost imperceptible with time. If a woman has a large frame or abundant fat around her jawline, she may require a couple more tiny incisions, on either side of the first one under the chin.

Many surgeons perform liposuction with their patients wide

awake and quite comfortable. I prefer my patients to be sedated or to have light general anesthesia during chin and neck liposuction, so that they feel no discomfort or anxiety while I'm working close to their faces.

Liposuctioning the chin, neck and jowls takes about an hour. The treated areas remain numb for one day after the procedure and anesthetic fluid drains from the tiny incision site during that time. Bruising and swelling are usually slight and mild pain killers generally suffice to control any discomfort. Patients are often surprised at how quickly they recover from tumescent liposuction; most return to light daily activities by the second or third day, and all but the most strenuous workouts can be resumed within a week of the procedure.

Patients achieve the best results by wearing a compression garment or girdle for a few weeks to a few months after liposuction; this optimizes skin re-contouring after the fat removal. (Several of my patients have termed it a "chin bra.") I like patients to wear this garment day and night for 3 to 5 days and then

for 10 to 12 hours a day for a month. Most patients can see improvement in their facial contours within a week of the procedure and all look significantly better after a month, although they often continue to improve for several months after this.

Many of my patients have described face and neck liposuction as a transformative experience. They don't just mean this in the physical sense—although removal of a double chin, sagging jowls or thickened neck certainly improves a face dramatically—but also in the psychological sense.

It is indescribably frustrating to struggle for years—and in vain—against genes that predestine you to develop fat deposits on your face, where there's no hope of hiding them. Patients frequently compare removal of this unwanted, and all too visible, fat to having a heavy burden lifted from their shoulders. And those who need to shape up elsewhere often become more motivated to do so once they are rid of this burden. As Serena, a 42-year-old financial planner, put it, "After my chin liposuction,

(continued)

Liposuction *(cont.)*

everyone kept telling me how good I looked now that I'd lost some weight. I guess they saw a slimmer face and equated it to a slimmer body. So I felt kind of inspired to start eating better and working out more!"

Safety demands that you insure your surgeon has the appropriate qualifications and experience. If he does, he will follow established safety guidelines, which limit the amount of numbing fluid you're given and the amount of fat that's removed in one session. And he'll insure that your sedation or general anesthesia, if you have either, is monitored properly. The liposuction horror stories you read or hear about are all avoidable—like the OB/GYN who performed liposuction on sedated patients in his office with no monitoring equipment and no anesthesiologist; or the inexperienced physician who took 8 hours to perform a liposuction that should have taken only 2, causing the patient to suffer huge fluid loss and anesthetic overdose.

As for the fat "all coming back," liposuction permanently removes fat cells and is a very effective treatment for problem areas that don't respond to a healthy diet and exercise. But it is not a cure for obesity. If you're more than 30 or 40 pounds overweight, it's better for you to establish a healthy eating and exercise regimen and at least start to lose weight before you consider liposuction. You won't tend to regain much fat in treated areas. But, if you gain a significant amount of weight, the fat will be deposited elsewhere. Your chin may no longer be the problem area that expands if you gain weight, but your waistline, arms or hips may instead. That's why the best candidate for liposuction is a woman who is already motivated to maintain a weight that's appropriate for her height and frame.

I've found that many of my patients benefit from consultation with a nutritionist and a personal trainer, both before and after their liposuction. A healthy diet and a regular fitness regimen allow them to maximize their results from liposuction.

Prominent skin pores become the bane of many a woman's existence as she ages. Sebum, the natural oil surrounding your hairs, tends to accumulate in your pores as your skin's cycle of renewal becomes less efficient. The sebum turns black when it's exposed to the air at your skin's surface, making your pores look darker and more noticeable. Your skin's decreasing resilience compounds this by making your sebum-filled pores gape open.

JoAnn, a kindergarten teacher in her early fifties, had struggled with this problem for years. She'd had several sessions of microdermabrasion—polishing of her skin with aluminum crystals—at another doctor's office, but to no avail.

"The kids in my class have started asking me why I have black spots on my nose," she sighed.

I recommended alternating sessions of salt macrodermabrasion and facials to JoAnn, but she was doubtful about the facials.

"I've had them before," she explained, "and all they did was inflame my skin because the beautician squeezed my blackheads so hard."

I started offering facials in my office precisely *because* so many women have had negative experiences. When properly performed, facials can work wonders for prominent pores by allowing the plugs of sebum that dilate them to be removed after gentle steaming. When I factor in the stress-reducing effects of facials too, I sometimes feel that they should be mandatory for all women seeking beautiful skin!

The trick is knowing where to go for your facials. I advise you to apply the same criteria that you would for choosing a cosmetic surgeon. Word-of-mouth is a useful place to start. Check the qualifications and experience of the person who'll be treating you, and talk to previous clients. And that sublime intangible, the magic touch, applies here too. Find an aesthetician or beautician who has it at her fingertips, and you're set.

If you're planning to have facials in a salon, rather than in a doctor's office, it's doubly important to check that everything that touches your skin is appropriately sanitized or sterilized, particularly if it's been in contact with other skin before yours. Otherwise, you're as much at risk of picking up infections from a facial as you are from sharing towels with a stranger. Emily is just one of several patients I've met who contracted impetigo—a highly infectious bacterial skin infection—from facials in salons. Fortunately, she came to see me as soon as she began to develop yellow-crusted patches on her face. Antibiotic pills saved her from the severe scarring that can occur if impetigo is not diagnosed and treated promptly.

In JoAnn's case, it took only one facial in my office to convince her that she was on the right track. After three sessions each of salt macrodermabrasion and facials, her pores were so improved that one of her small students actually asked her where her black spots had gone.

Are "Lunchtime Procedures" Still the Flavor of the Month?

A few years back, "lunchtime" procedures—cosmetic surgery that requires little or no recovery time—were hot and happening. Some even predicted that these procedures would supersede traditional cosmetic surgery requiring downtime. Why, the argument went, would a woman choose to look like a skinned tomato for a week or two after laser resurfacing when she could zap her wrinkles with the NLite or CoolTouch laser, put on her makeup, walk out the door, and go straight back to her regular daily activities?

To some extent, this prediction has come true. Many of the procedures I'm discussing with you qualify as lunchtime procedures. And many of my patients do zip down to my office on their lunch breaks, often to have several procedures at one sitting. For instance, Meg, a 47-year-old financial analyst, routinely drives to my office from hers for salt macrodermabrasion of her face, collagen injections of her lips and smile lines, eyebrow shaping, and Botox injections of her frown lines, and is back at her desk with time to spare.

Lunchtime procedures have definitely made cosmetic surgery more accessible to those who have to work for a living or simply have limited time on their hands. But along with their increasing popularity has come the realization that they are not a panacea for every aging woe. Unfortunately, some women attain that realization only after the fact: when a procedure their doctor wholeheartedly recommended or they avidly sought themselves after hearing the latest buzz fails to deliver the goods. This letdown has led to something of a backlash against lunchtime procedures, from patients—and from physicians.

At a recent medical conference, a well-known dermatologist told me, "I'm not very impressed with CoolTouch; about half my patients are unhappy with their results."

When I inquired further, I learned that this physician spent little time actually discussing the laser procedure with his patients. He would mention it by name and leave the exam room. His assistant would then discuss the procedure with the patient, emphasizing the fees involved, and book the first appointment.

This approach is practically a guaranteed setup for dissatisfied patients because it overlooks one important point about many lunchtime procedures. The trade-off for no recovery time is that your results are compromised to some extent. For instance, the CoolTouch laser can remove your wrinkles and scars to almost the same degree as laser resurfacing—in experienced hands. But what it won't do is tighten skin or fade discolorations the way that laser resurfacing does.

Now, imagine you visited a doctor, seeking to rejuvenate your eyes. If he recommended the CoolTouch laser without any further discussion, you might reasonably expect it to not only improve your crow's-feet but also fade your dark under-eye circles and tighten your droopy eyelids. And you might reasonably be disappointed when it didn't.

Botox and collagen injections have their trade-offs too, not in the results but in how long the results last. If it's not explained to you that these treatments have to be repeated two or three times a year, you're going to be pretty disillusioned. I've certainly met patients whose doctors didn't apprise them of this vital fact.

It can be tempting to treat lunchtime procedures as "cosmetic surgery lite," as if minimal recovery time equaled minimal emotional investment in the procedures themselves or in the doctor–patient relationship. But that's a temptation both you and your doctor should resist. To my mind, it's doubly important for a physician to establish good rapport with you if he's discussing lunchtime procedures. That's the only way he can fully understand your expectations and gauge how close a procedure can come to meeting them. If you would be quite happy with less dramatic results in the interests of no recovery time, then lunchtime procedures are the way to go. If you wouldn't, then they're not.

(continued on page 258)

Lunchtime Lasers

Lasers that soften your lines or re-move spider veins or sunspots with little or no recovery time have revolutionized cosmetic surgery . . . and demolished the "no pain, no gain" dictum. No lunchtime laser can give you the dramatic skin tightening or wrinkle removal that laser resur-facing or medium chemical peeling can. But they can produce quite im-pressive results in the hands of a physician who thoroughly under-stands laser technology. And they can be used safely on skin of all colors.

The two lasers that I prefer for improvement of wrinkles and scars are the NLite and the CoolTouch. Both work by stimulating your skin to produce new collagen. Over a se-ries of three to five sessions (some-times more for CoolTouch), spaced 2 to 4 weeks apart, targeted treatment around the eyes or mouth can signif-icantly reduce crows feet and fine upper lip wrinkles. Treatment can be performed elsewhere on the face to soften shallow acne and chickenpox scars. Each session takes about 15 to 30 minutes and you will experience mild stinging each time the laser

beam is applied to your skin. Many of my patients use numbing cream before treatment so that they barely feel any discomfort, although some find treatment quite tolerable even without numbing.

These are not instant gratification procedures. Immediately after treat-ment, all you'll be aware of is mild flushing or pinkness, which usually fades within an hour or two. As with all lunchtime procedures, you can apply makeup and resume reg-ular activities right after an NLite or CoolTouch session. But it takes time and cumulative treatments for your skin to produce enough collagen for you to see significant results. My patients usually begin to notice im-provement 6 weeks or so after their first session, by which time they have already returned for their second or third treatment. Because of the lag time between treatment and collagen formation, your skin may continue to improve for several months after your last session. NLite or CoolTouch treatment costs a few hundred dollars per session for each area treated and discount packages are often available.

I believe that the key to success with lunchtime wrinkle lasers is to insure that patients understand clearly what these lasers can achieve . . . and what they cannot. And, as with all lasers, it's vital for your cosmetic surgeon to have in-depth knowledge of laser science. Laser surgery, whether lunchtime or traditional, is a finely balanced art. The surgeon must select settings for the laser energy, duration of laser pulses and time between them—to name just a few variables—to maximize results and minimize side effects. If the settings are too high you may get results—but at the cost of skin irritation or even scarring. If the settings are too low, you'll be correspondingly "underwhelmed" with the results. I've found I can get lunchtime wrinkle lasers to work best for my patients by doing what I call "pushing the parameters". This means that I treat aggressively to the point of skin pinkness but always take care not to go beyond this point and cause skin blistering or scabbing.

My laser of choice for spider veins and other red spots, and also for sunspots, is the Diolite laser. It produces a concentrated yellow-green laser beam which targets either blood or melanin pigment,

depending on what the laser is aimed at. The resultant heat instantly destroys the target without damaging the surrounding skin. The big innovation of the Diolite and similar lasers is that they do not cause any bruising after treatment and thus they are truly lunchtime lasers. They cause skin pinkness for a few hours to a few days in the areas where spider veins or red spots have been removed but this can be covered up with makeup straight after the procedure. Treated sunspots and freckles tend to darken slightly for a week or so after treatment, before they flake off, leaving slightly pink areas which fade within a few weeks. One session of treatment, lasting 15 to 30 minutes and costing a few hundred dollars, may be all that's needed to treat your whole face. If additional sessions are needed, they may be at a reduced price. I occasionally use the more traditional pulse dye laser for larger collections of blood vessels, such as those in a birthmark. Although this laser does cause bruising after treatment, it often lasts only a few days with the newer pulse dye lasers.

Another type of lunchtime skin treatment is known as **intense**

(continued)

Lunchtime Lasers *(cont.)*

pulsed light (IPL) therapy and marketed under the brand names, Foto-Facial, Photorejuvenation and Epifacial. A true laser produces an intense light beam of only one color or wavelength. IPL is not truly a laser treatment because it employs a light beam of multiple wavelengths. This feature of IPL is touted by the manufacturers as contributing to its flexibility; a physician who consults for one of these manufacturers once told me poetically that IPL is like "painting all the colors of the rainbow". But reality is rather more prosaic. The multiple wavelengths of IPL make it less selective; a laser has one single target whereas IPL has several. This may not be a problem on the lightest skin, where IPL has the potential to treat wrinkles, spider veins and sunspots simultaneously, albeit non-selectively. But IPL can be a disaster on skin which is even slightly olive-toned, let alone more pigmented, as it readily causes skin discolorations which may be quite difficult to fade. Whatever the skin type of my patients, I prefer to use separate, true lasers to treat separate conditions. That way, I can individualize each laser's settings and achieve the fine control that I feel is necessary for the best results—rather than using one blanket setting to treat a collection of unrelated skin problems.

You should also keep in mind that lunchtime procedures generally require several sessions of treatment, as opposed to traditional cosmetic surgery, which tends to be a "one-shot deal." Both types of surgery may end up costing you almost the same, the difference being that you pay that cost all at once with traditional surgery but pay it by the session with a lunchtime procedure.

The backlash against lunchtime procedures was perhaps inevitable, given the hype of the past few years. But it's throwing the baby out with the bathwater to blame the procedures when we should be blaming poor communication between physicians and patients. My own experience with lunchtime procedures has been overwhelmingly positive. Meg is just one of my many patients who is extremely happy with her results. And she's pointed out to me that she could never have had surgery requiring downtime, given the demands of her personal and professional life.

How Long Will Your Results Last?

If you're trying to figure out whether a procedure is worth it for you, or trying to choose between procedures, this is an all-important question. And it's easy to answer for some procedures. On average, Botox and collagen treatments wear off and need repeating every 3 to 6 months. If you find that off-putting, consider the fact that you'd never have a haircut, take a shower, or cut your toenails if you eschewed all things temporary.

For other procedures, the question is a little more complicated. Eva, who's 53, confidently reported that "another doctor told me my chemical peel would last 7 years." But that's the medical equivalent of quantifying how long it'll take you to feel hungry again after you eat a cheese sandwich. In reality, there's only one answer for procedures of this type: "It all depends."

Ultimately, we're not really talking about how long a result *lasts*. Remove the uppermost layer of your epidermis with a chemical peel, and, technically speaking, the effect lasts forever because those particular skin cells were permanently removed.

What most women really mean when they ask "How long will my results last?" is "How long will it take for me to look old again?" or "How long will it be before I need to repeat the procedure?" And that all depends on how fast you age. If you've damaged your skin with too much sun, smoke, stress, or the like in the years before your procedure, your surgery may reverse some, but not all, of this. Any damage that remains will increase your aging rate after the surgery.

And of course if you continue the damage after surgery, the outlook is worse. Bonnie's laser resurfacing of her neck and chest lasted only 2 months—until she went out on her boat all day without sunscreen on her neck and chest and got burned. I had to redo her whole procedure to get rid of the resultant sunspots. Contrast this with her face, which I'd also lasered. She protected it with sunscreen and makeup on that ill-fated day, and it still looks great 5 years after her procedure.

A rejuvenating procedure turns back your aging clock but cannot stop its ticking. When we speak of a face-lift's "dropping" after a certain number of years, that's a misconception. Your face starts to sag again not because your face-lift wore off but because you've continued to age. The truth is, no cosmetic surgery is permanent because aging cannot be stopped.

Even if you can't precisely predict how fast you'll age after surgery, there is one thing you can predict. With any procedure that's properly performed, you'll always look better than if you hadn't had it done. And don't forget: the more careful you are with your skin after your procedure, the slower your aging clock will tick.

Dollars and Sense

You've defined your problems, found the right cosmetic surgeon, figured out what procedures you want and are ready to go. But there's one last consideration that you shouldn't overlook, and that's the bottom line. Before you schedule your appointment, make sure you clarify with your doctor or his staff precisely what you'll be paying. As indelicate as this may seem at the time, it's the only way you can avoid misunderstandings in the future. Each office has its own pricing policies and it's imperative that you understand those of the office you've chosen for your treatment.

Many offices provide you with a written financial agreement, which should state explicitly what and when you need to pay for your surgery. This agreement should also indicate if you are required to put down an advance deposit. In my office, for example, patients pay 50 percent of their procedure fee in advance when they schedule all but the most minor procedures. Make sure you understand whether the fee you see in the agreement is the total you will pay, or whether there are additional costs. The most common additional costs are for surgical supplies (such as special skin dressings after laser surgery or compression garments to be worn after liposuction) and for the anesthesiologist, if one is required for your procedure.

The financial agreement should also clarify the office's cancellation policy. How much notice do you have to give when cancelling your appointment and, if you don't give enough notice, will you forfeit part or all of your deposit? Keep in mind that the overhead for many procedures is substantial. For instance, if you call and cancel your liposuction only a few hours before it's due to occur, it's likely that significant manpower and supplies will already have been expended to prepare for your procedure. In addition, the surgeon and the anesthesiologist will have blocked out several hours of time for you, during which they could have been treating other patients. The office or surgical center may have to retain your deposit to cover this overhead.

You may particularly need to clarify the office's policy regarding so-called "touch-up" treatments. If you have a procedure that gives you partial results and the procedure needs to be performed again at some later date for full results, this is known as a touch-up treatment. If you buy a package of five hair laser treatments and then it turns out that you need a sixth to leave your upper lip fuzz-free, do you pay full price, reduced price or nothing at all for it? If you need a little more Botox to smooth your frown lines totally, 1 week after your first treatment removed most of them, what will be the fee? How about if the Botox touch-up is a month later? It's best to know what to expect before you embark on treatment. That way, you can relax and enjoy the results of your surgery. And your doctor can be fully focused on giving you these results, not on paperwork or other red tape.

The Transformation of Hannah

Of all my patients, Hannah's the one who never fails to bring *The Rose Geranium* to my mind. A homemaker and busy charity volunteer in her mid-fifties, she first came to see me a few weeks after another physician's nurse had treated her with collagen injections.

"I've spent thousands of dollars on collagen, Botox, and chemical peels," she told me, "and I don't look any better. In fact, if you ask me, I look worse."

Looking at Hannah's face, I had to agree. The collagen injections had been placed just a fraction of an inch too high, forming a ridge that only made her smile lines appear deeper.

"All my treatment's been so piecemeal: a little collagen here, a little Botox there," Hannah continued. "I want you to give me an overall plan."

My plan for Hannah was to strengthen her power points, which had been totally neglected in all the work she'd had done so far. Her skin was in pretty good shape, apart from the sunspots that detracted from its clarity. Her eyebrows were a waxing disaster—they were low and flat and gave her a look of permanent annoyance. And her mouth, which she told me had never been full even in its heyday, had now thinned to the extent that her upper lip was virtually invisible.

(continued on page 267)

Permanent Makeup

Permanent makeup sounds like a dream come true for any busy woman on the go. What could be better than not having to waste precious minutes putting on your "face" every morning; or not having to contend with the "raccoon eyes" of smudged eyeliner after a swimming session or readjustment of a wayward contact lens?

Unfortunately, reality is not so simple. Permanent makeup is actually cosmetic tattooing; pigment is embedded within the skin using tiny needles. Numbing cream is often used to lessen discomfort during this process, which may take several sessions. The procedure used to apply permanent eyeliner, eyebrow color, blusher or lip liner to your face is exactly the same as that used for the tattoos with which you may be more familiar. And the same risks apply too.

A couple of years ago, I stopped by a beauty salon that advertised permanent makeup. I was shocked to hear the owner tell me that she possessed only one tattooing needle, which she boiled in water and then re-used, because it was too expensive to provide

sterile, disposable needles for each client. I explained to the hairdresser in no uncertain terms that boiling water does not sterilize a needle adequately and that she was putting her clients at risk of infectious diseases, including viral hepatitis, AIDS and bacterial infections. I hope she got the message.

If you decide to have permanent makeup applied after reading the information here, please make sure the procedure is done in a qualified physician's office, by the physician herself or by an experienced assistant. Ideally, both the tattoo needles and the containers of pigment should be new and sterile for each patient. That way, there's no risk that you'll be exposed to another patient's infections through "double-dipping" of a needle into a pigment container.

Cosmetic tattooing carries aesthetic risks too, as Claudine, a lithe and athletic ski instructor in her mid-sixties, discovered. She had always been unhappy with her thin lips, and she became more so as the years went by and the vertical wrinkles on her upper lip deepened. She had permanent lip liner applied by a cosmetic tattooist who advertised extensively. Claudine was disappointed right after the procedure because the lip liner was not the subtle flesh tone she'd been promised, but a garish orange-pink. Far from being able to throw away her makeup, she now felt obliged to wear lipstick constantly to camouflage her permanent lip liner.

By the time Claudine came to see me 4 years after the tattooing, the pigment had migrated away from her natural lip line and onto the skin of her upper lip, an effect that was compounded by continued thinning of her lips with age. The permanent lip line resembled a thin, peach-colored mustache penciled above her lip. She asked if a laser could remove it, but I shook my head. Lasers work quite well for removing the black or brown pigments that are used for permanent eyeliner and eyebrow shading. But there's a significant risk that a pink, pale brown or orange tattoo may turn intensely black after laser treatment. The tattoo is then more disfiguring and may be impossible to remove.

The solution I proposed was to leave the tattoo in place but to correct the thinning and wrinkling of Claudine's lips, which was what she had been trying to fix originally. I accomplished this with fat injections and, in doing so, raised her natural lip line so that the tattoo lay over it.

Claudine was extremely happy with the result, as the tattoo was now barely visible and she no longer had to wear lipstick to conceal it.

Permanent eyeliner is even more likely to move away from where it's placed, resulting in permanent raccoon eyes. In my opinion, the only place it's worth considering this procedure is for your eyebrows . . . if they've become virtually non-existent due to years of over-plucking or as a result of injury. Eyebrow tattoos don't look particularly natural, but they're preferable to the unattractive alternative of going eyebrow-less.

I believe the vogue for permanent makeup is, to some extent, a reflection of obsession with perfection. It reinforces the concept that a woman should look immaculate from the moment she wakes up until the moment she retires to bed in her designer negligee. But, to me, there's something harsh and unappealing about eyeliner that never blurs or lips that remain immutably defined. My aunt, now in her eighties but still as mentally agile as ever, has always said that makeup looks best when it's not quite perfect, but is softened by a little smudging. She'd have made a great cosmetic surgeon!

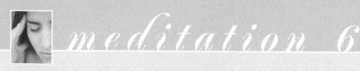

Visualizing Your Face at Different Ages and Seeing the Changes Positively

This meditation builds upon Meditations 3 and 4 ("Seeing Your Face Positively" I on page 92 and II on page 96). With the aid of photographs, you will visualize the specific aging changes that have occurred in your face. You will acknowledge the changes that make you appear older, but you'll focus on the positive changes of time—and there are always some. Again, this meditation may arouse feelings of discomfort because our youth-oriented culture has ingrained in us the belief that aging is a negative process.

Your discomfort can be allayed by visualizing your inner beauty as a protective shield of light and warmth. As you practice this meditation, you will begin to appreciate the increased potential for wisdom and spirituality that you gain as you age.

You will need a photograph of your face at the age of about 18 and a photograph for every 5 to 10 years since then. You should have three to six photographs. Before you begin, lay out the photos in chronological order in front of you so that you can see them with your head in a relaxed position.

1. Sit comfortably in a quiet place, with your back straight. Your head should be in an unstrained, neutral position. Rest your hands in your lap or clasp them together lightly, and place your legs in a comfortable resting position.

2. Close your eyes gently.

3. Inhale slowly and deeply through your nose while mentally counting to 10.

4. Exhale slowly and fully through your mouth while mentally counting to 10. Feel yourself becoming aware of the thoughts that are passing through your mind.

5. Visualize your thoughts moving across your mind from left to right like a billowing stream of white smoke. Observe how the speed and density of the smoke vary with time; this represents your ever-changing thoughts.

6. Continue to inhale slowly and deeply through your nose again and exhale slowly through your mouth while continuing to focus on the stream of smoke. While doing this, repeat to yourself, "I am at peace."

7. Repeat the inhaling and exhaling until you have achieved an effortless breathing rhythm and feel a sense of serenity enveloping you.

8. Feel yourself moving closer and closer to the smoke and finally passing through it.

9. Visualize a constant, glowing orange-red flame behind the smoke screen. This represents your Self: your here-and-now feeling of being or existing.

10. Continue to breathe slowly and deeply until you have achieved an effortless breathing pattern and are no longer aware of the smoke, but only of the flame.

11. Feel the flame's light and warmth radiating toward you. This represents your consciousness: the life and energy that emanates from your Self.

12. Continue to breathe effortlessly while focusing on the flame and its light and warmth. Feel yourself moving toward the flame and your mind being pulled in toward it.

13. When you feel a sense of serenity enveloping you, focus on it for at least 10 seconds. Then open your eyes slowly.

14. Look at each photograph in turn for at least 10 seconds, noting the changes in your face that have occurred with age. Examine your eyes and the skin around them, your mouth and surrounding areas, and then the rest of your

Continued on page 266

face. When examining the photographs, try to do so objectively, as if they were of another person.

15. Now look in the mirror at your face and examine each area in turn. If you begin to experience negative feelings about your appearance or feel uneasy during the self-appraisal, repeat steps 3 and 4 until the feeling of calmness returns.

16. Note the changes between your face now and previously. First, focus upon signs of aging—wrinkles, discolorations or age spots, spider veins, or loose skin. Try to be objective when performing this self-appraisal. Continue to breathe slowly and deeply.

17. Now focus upon the positive changes in your face, such as the wisdom or serenity in your eyes, the increased warmth of your smile, or the accentuation of your bone structure.

18. Close your eyes and visualize the progression of the aging changes you see in your face. Maintain a feeling of calmness and objectivity as you do so, and continue to breathe slowly and deeply.

19. Place your fingertips lightly on your temples, and visualize your inner beauty as a stream of light and warmth emanating from the flame within you through your pupils and from a flame at the base of your spine. Visualize the stream of light and warmth enveloping you in beauty.

20. Continue to breathe slowly and deeply. When you feel a sense of clarity and serenity, open your eyes slowly.

By the time Hannah attended her next charity ball, I'd taken care of her sunspots with the Diolite laser and injected her lips with her own fat, plus a layer of collagen over that for definition. Her eyebrows were in better shape, but years of waxing had slowed their growth and it would take another couple of months before they grew out sufficiently for perfect arching. Hannah's previous experience with Botox had not been good. It had relaxed the wrinkles on her forehead but it also made her eyelids feel—and look—heavy for months afterward. I re-treated her with the utmost caution, avoiding the areas I knew would lower her eyelids and injecting a little Botox just above the highest point of her eyebrows to raise them and relieve any eyelid heaviness.

When I was done, even I was a little overwhelmed at the results. Hannah's face had looked pinched and defeated before. Now there was so much to enjoy in her extravagantly lashed hazel eyes, high cheekbones, and creamy complexion. I thought back to her first visit 2 months previously. And I saw changes that extended far beyond her face, in the light that radiated from within her eyes and in her warm, confident smile. Even her wardrobe had metamorphosed: She'd gone from earth-toned slacks to snappy, above-the-knee outfits in primary colors.

As she strode into the waiting room and waved to my staff, another patient spoke my thoughts aloud: "Now, there's a woman who feels beautiful!"

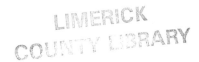

Epilogue

Making Peace
with Aging

We are always the same age inside.

—Gertrude Stein

ood genes, a healthy lifestyle, and skillful beauty enhancement can slow the clock of aging, but they cannot stop its ticking. It's difficult to age gracefully and fearlessly when society bombards us with the message that youth and physical beauty—the most transient of our attributes—are everything.

Fortunately, most of us have role models for aging with grace, maybe a friend or a relative who appears to grow more contented with age. My mother and aunts are inspirations to me—they continue to live young by exercising, playing music, meditating, and, most of all, keeping their minds active. They remind me that age is measured not in years or wrinkles but in accumulated life wisdom; they remind me that the beauty that dwells inside us is ageless and ever radiant.

Aging with grace means different things to different people. One of my physician colleagues began to go gray in her twenties and was completely white-haired by her late thirties. It's not just the stunningly beautiful contrast between her hair and her olive skin that turns heads when she walks down the street. It's also her air of complete comfort with herself.

Contrast this with Norma, a spiritual and healthy-living 67-year-old. For years, she'd looked much younger than her actual age. And she was devastated when she experienced a sudden spurt of aging and people suddenly began to peg her as a senior citizen. For Norma, feeling consistently unhappy about how she looked was not what she considered aging gracefully. I injected fat into the furrows around her mouth, treated her frown lines with Botox, and tightened her jawline and faded her sunspots with chemical peels. These treatments restored the balance between how she felt inside and how she looked outside and, together with her inner strength, allowed her to feel at peace.

Making peace with aging is one of the most challenging parts of being human because it means acknowledging the transience of our bodies and, hopefully, embracing the eternity of our souls. You have every right to pursue and achieve the outward manifestation of the beauty that lies within you. But peace is possible only when you believe that the seat of your beauty, your inner beauty, improves with age and never dies. When you face up to the inevitability—and the spiritual magnificence—of aging, then you can truly value the woman you are, and the woman you will become.

meditation 7

Reuniting Your Inner and Outer Beauty

This, the final meditation, incorporates and expands upon elements of the previous meditations. You will invoke the vision of your inner Self as a flame radiating light and warmth that represent your inner beauty. You will recall the positive image of your face and visualize your inner beauty radiating outward as light and warmth breaking through its barrier and enveloping your external persona. You will also visualize your life force rising as light and warmth from the base of your spine.

With practice, you will be able to visualize the uniting of your inner and outer beauty even when you are not in a complete meditative state. Your face will become the mirror of your soul, reflecting the luminosity of serenity, confidence, compassion, and self-esteem.

1. Sit comfortably in a quiet place, with your back straight. Your head should be in an unstrained, neutral position. Rest your hands in your lap or clasp them together lightly, and place your legs in a comfortable resting position.

2. Close your eyes gently.

3. Inhale slowly and deeply through your nose while mentally counting to 10.

4. Exhale slowly and fully through your mouth while mentally counting to 10. Feel yourself becoming aware of the thoughts that are passing through your mind.

5. Visualize your thoughts moving across your mind from left to right like a billowing stream of white smoke. Observe how the speed and density of the smoke vary with time; this represents your ever-changing thoughts.

6. Continue to inhale slowly and deeply through your nose again and exhale slowly through your mouth while continuing to focus on the stream of smoke. While doing this, repeat to yourself, "I am at peace."

7. Repeat the inhaling and exhaling until you have achieved an effortless breathing rhythm and feel a sense of serenity enveloping you.

8. Feel yourself moving closer to the smoke and finally passing through it.

9. Visualize a constant, glowing orange-red flame behind the smoke screen. This represents your Self: your here-and-now feeling of being or existing.

10. Feel the flame's light and warmth radiating toward you.

11. Continue to breathe effortlessly while focusing on the flame and its light and warmth. Feel yourself moving toward the flame and your mind being pulled in toward it.

12. When you feel a sense of serenity enveloping you, focus on it for at least 10 seconds. Then open your eyes slowly.

13. Examine your eyes and the skin around them, your mouth and surrounding areas, and then the rest of your face. Continue to breathe slowly and deeply.

14. Close your eyes. Place your hands lightly on your face so that your fingertips span your forehead. With slow, gentle sweeping motions, touch your face and neck, concentrating on the texture, softness, and warmth of your skin. Touch the curve of your cheekbones, nose, and chin; the curve of your eyebrows and lips; your earlobes and your neck. As you feel each area, recall the visual memory of it, and inhale and continue to breathe slowly and deeply.

15. Visualize your inner beauty as a stream of light and warmth projecting from the flame within you through your pupils and from a flame at the base of your spine. As you continue to sweep your fingertips across your face, visualize the streams of light and warmth enveloping and protecting it.

16. Place your fingertips lightly on your temples. Visualize the progression of aging changes in your face. Visualize the streams of light and warmth breaking across the surface of your whole face and spreading within and throughout it.

17. Visualize your face glowing with light and warmth. Continue to breathe slowly and deeply. When you feel an overwhelming sense of clarity, confidence, and serenity, slowly open your eyes.

Credits

"*Que Será, Será*" by Jay Livingston and Raymond B. Evans, on page 1. Copyright © 1955, renewed 1984 Universal-MCA Music Publishing on behalf of St. Angelo Music. All rights reserved. Used by permission.

The Goldie Hawn quotation on page 22 is reprinted from the article "Celebrity Surgery" by Dorota Nosowitz, *The Observer,* August 2000. Reprinted with permission. © 2000 *The Observer.*

Excerpt from the poem "Binker" on page 50 from *Now We Are Six* by A. A. Milne, illustrated by E. H. Shepard, copyright 1927 by E. P. Dutton, renewed © 1955 by A. A. Milne. Used by permission of Dutton Children's Books, A division of Penguin Young Readers Group, A Member of Penguin Group (USA) Inc., 345 Hudson Street, New York, NY 10014. All rights reserved. Reprinted with permission.

The Anaïs Nin quotation on page 68 is reprinted from *The Diary of Anaïs Nin 1939–1944, Volume III*, Harcourt, Inc., 1971. Reprinted with permission.

The Anne Lamott quotation on page 77 is reprinted from *Bird by Bird*, by Anne Lamott, Anchor Books, 1994. Reprinted with permission.

The Jean Kerr quotation on page 109 is reprinted from *The Snake Has All the Lines*. Doubleday, Division of Random House, 1960. Reprinted with permission.

The Albert Einstein quotation on page 147 is reprinted from *Albert Einstein's Autobiographical Notes*, Open Court Publishing Company, 1979. Reprinted with permission.

The Arthur C. Clarke quotation on page 217 is reprinted from *Profiles of the Future*, Henry Holt and Company, 1962. Revised edition: Victor Gollancz, 1999. Reprinted with the author's permission.

Index

Underscored page references indicate boxed text.